JN237257

ティアニー先生の
ベスト・パール

The Best
Clinical Pearls
of Dr. Tierney

ティアニー先生の
ベスト・パール

ローレンス・ティアニー
Lawrence M. Tierney Jr.
カリフォルニア大学サンフランシスコ校内科学教授

訳・**松村正巳**
Masami Matsumura
金沢大学医学教育研究センター准教授
リウマチ・膠原病内科

The Best
Clinical Pearls
of Dr. Tierney

医学書院

ティアニー先生のベスト・パール

発　行	2011年10月15日　第1版第1刷 ©
著　者	ローレンス・ティアニー
訳　者	松村正巳 _{まつむらまさみ}
発行者	株式会社　医学書院 　　代表取締役　金原　優 　　〒113-8719　東京都文京区本郷 1-28-23 　　電話　03-3817-5600（社内案内）

印刷・製本　三美印刷

本書の複製権・翻訳権・上映権・譲渡権・公衆送信権（送信可能化権を含む）
は㈱医学書院が保有します．

ISBN978-4-260-01465-6

本書を無断で複製する行為（複写，スキャン，デジタルデータ化など）は，「私的使用のための複製」など著作権法上の限られた例外を除き禁じられています．大学，病院，診療所，企業などにおいて，業務上使用する目的（診療，研究活動を含む）で上記の行為を行うことは，その使用範囲が内部的であっても，私的使用には該当せず，違法です．また私的使用に該当する場合であっても，代行業者等の第三者に依頼して上記の行為を行うことは違法となります．

JCOPY　〈㈳出版者著作権管理機構　委託出版物〉
本書の無断複写は著作権法上での例外を除き禁じられています．複写される場合は，そのつど事前に，㈳出版者著作権管理機構（電話 03-3513-6969，FAX 03-3513-6979，info@jcopy.or.jp）の許諾を得てください．

序 — PREFACE

　私たちは読者の方々に，まだ完結していないこのパール集を楽しんでいただけるものと期待しています．そして，この本が読者にとって興味深いものであれば，続編を出版したいと考えています．大切なことは，パールとは，本書に記されているような表現形式によって，医学における絶対的な確信を示すものであることを知っていただくことです．よく知られているように，医学において100％正しいということはありません．本書に付した，それぞれのパールの解説を読むことにより，医学生や研修医，臨床医のみなさんが各パールの意味するところのものを，より的確に理解していただけるのではないかと期待しています．

　「パール」という名称が慣用的に使われるようになったのは，何年も前に遡ります．40年以上前に私が医学生だった頃から「パール」と呼ばれていたことをよく覚えています．また，パールは短く，記憶しやすい限り，とても優れた教育ツールだと考えられています．これはさらに詳細な，エビデンスに基づいた臨床診断の解析の放棄を意味するものではありません．医学を学ぶすべての人は，個人的な経験，医学雑誌，教科書，世代から世代へ受け継がれるパールなどを含む，いくつもの方法で学ぶことが大切なのです．パールの歴史という話題は，あるいは，医学雑誌の目を引く記事になるかもしれません．しかし実際には，この用語がいつ生まれたのかを特定するのは困難でしょう．一つ確かなことは，パールとは，教える者と学ぶ者の関係のなかで，世界中に広まるものだということです．これは私の経験から間違いのないことだと言えます．

　この本では，私たちの知る限りこれまでにはなかった，英語で書かれたパールとその解説をほかの言語へ翻訳することを試みました．本書の場合には日本語への翻訳です．おそらく，読者の方々には，パールの包含する概念をより深く理解していただけるでしょう．あるパールでは，直接的に，英語での流れ・語感のほうが理解してもらうのにふさわしいでしょう．一方で，日本語に訳されたパールのほうがよりよいという場合もあるでしょう．

　言うまでもないことですが，私たちの目的は，言語にかかわらず，どんな方法であろうと医学の学びへの情熱を刺激することです．この本が読者に興味をもたらすであろうことを心から願っています．

The authors hope that readers enjoy this collection of clinical pearls, which is by no means complete, and indeed, we hope that if it proves to be of interest, another volume might be published. It is important to recognize that clinical pearls are stated in such a way as to suggest absolute certainty of content; in medicine, it is well-known that nothing is 100%, and thus, it is hoped the explanations of the pearls may allow students, residents, and practicing physicians to understand the meaning more clearly. The usage of the term "Pearl" goes back many years; one of the authors (LT) well remembers them being stated as such during his years in medical school more than 40 years ago. It is also the impression of the authors that the clinical pearl is an excellent teaching tool insofar as it is short, and easier to remember. This is not to suggest that more detailed, evidence-based analysis of clinical diagnoses be abandoned; far from it. It is crucial that as students of medicine, we all learn in several ways, including personal experience, medical journals and textbooks, and the clinical pearls which are handed down from generation to generation. Indeed, the history of the clinical pearl might well make for an amusing article in a journal, but we suspect it would be difficult to determine when this terminology came into being. One thing is certain: it is widespread throughout the world among teachers and students, as can be attested by experience of the authors.

This volume attempts something that has not been tried before to our knowledge, namely, the translation of pearls and their explanations from English into another language, in this case, Japanese, so the reader might be able better to understand the concept the pearl entails. In certain cases, simply the flow of the English language, and its qualities of sound, may make it more appropriate in that language; in other instances, perhaps the Japanese pearl is better than the English. No matter: it is our aim to stimulate enthusiasm for learning medicine in any fashion, and we truly hope that this book will be of interest to the readership.

2011年9月
September, 2011

ローレンス・ティアニー
Lawrence M. Tierney Jr, MD

松村正巳（訳）
Masami Matsumura, MD

CONTENTS
目次

VASCULAR DISEASES　　　001
血管性疾患

1. Angina Pectoris
   狭心症
2. Aortic Dissection
   大動脈解離
3. Aortic Coarctation
   大動脈縮窄症
4. Aortic Insufficiency
   大動脈弁閉鎖不全
5. Aortic Stenosis
   大動脈弁狭窄
6. Mitral Stenosis
   僧帽弁狭窄
7. Mitral Regurgitation
   僧帽弁閉鎖不全
8. Atrial Fibrillation
   心房細動
9. Atrial Flutter
   心房粗動
10. Atrial Septal Defect
    心房中隔欠損症
11. Congestive Heart Failure
    うっ血性心不全
12. Constrictive Pericarditis
    収縮性心膜炎
13. Hypertension
    高血圧症
14. Ventricular Tachycardia
    心室頻拍

INFECTIOUS DISEASES   017
感染症

15. Brucellosis
    ブルセラ症

16. Cat Scratch Disease
    ネコひっかき病

17. Cholera
    コレラ

18. Typhoid Fever
    腸チフス

19. Leprosy
    ハンセン病

20. Leptospirosis
    レプトスピラ症

21. Bacterial Meningitis
    細菌性髄膜炎

22. Pertussis
    百日咳

23. Pneumococcal Infections
    肺炎球菌感染症

24. Streptococcal Pharyngitis
    連鎖球菌咽頭炎

25. Primary Syphilis
    第1期梅毒

26. Secondary Syphilis
    第2期梅毒

27. Tuberculosis
    結核

28. Coccidiomycosis
    コクシジオイデス症

29. Cryptococcosis
    クリプトコッカス症

30. Histoplasmosis
    ヒストプラズマ症

31. Pneumocystis Pneumonia (PCP)
    ニューモシスチス肺炎

32. Cysticercosis
    嚢虫症

33. Schistosomiasis
    ヒト住血吸虫症

34. Strongyloidiasis
    糞線虫症

35. Fish Tapeworm
    広節裂頭条虫

36. Amoebiasis
    アメーバ症

37. Trypanosomiasis (Chagas' Disease)
    トリパノソーマ症

38. Visceral Leishmaniasis
    内臓型リーシュマニア症

39. Q Fever
    Q熱

40. Tsutsugamushi Disease
    ツツガムシ病

41. Cytomegalovirus Disease
    サイトメガロウイルス感染症

42. HIV Infection
    HIV感染症

43. Multiple Sclerosis
    多発性硬化症

NEOPLASTIC DISEASES
腫瘍性疾患
047

44. Breast Cancer
乳癌

45. Central Nervous System Tumors
中枢神経腫瘍

46. Cervical Cancer
子宮頸癌

47. Colon Cancer
大腸癌

48. Esophageal Cancer
食道癌

49. Gastric Carcinoma
胃癌

50. Gestational Trophoblastic Neoplasia
妊娠性栄養膜新生物

51. Hepatocellular Carcinoma
肝細胞癌

52. Lung Cancer
肺癌

53. Prostate Cancer
前立腺癌

54. Renal Cell Carcinoma
腎細胞癌

55. Testicular Cancer
精巣癌

HEMATOLOGIC TUMORS
血液悪性腫瘍
061

56. Acute Leukemia
急性白血病

57. Chronic Lymphocytic Leukemia
慢性リンパ性白血病

58. Chronic Myelogenous Leukemia
慢性骨髄性白血病

59. Essential Thrombocytosis
本態性血小板増加症

60. Hodgkin's Disease
ホジキン病

61. Multiple Myeloma
多発性骨髄腫

62. Non-Hodgkin's Lymphoma
非ホジキンリンパ腫

63. Paroxysmal Nocturnal Hemoglobinuria
発作性夜間ヘモグロビン尿症

64. Polycythemia Vera
真性赤血球症

65. Waldenström's Macroglobulinemia
マクログロブリン血症

RHEUMATOLOGY　　　　073
自己免疫性疾患

66. Adult Still's Disease
    成人スティル病
67. Ankylosing Spondylitis
    強直性脊椎炎
68. Arthritis Associated with Inflammatory Bowel Disease
    炎症性腸疾患に伴う関節炎
69. Behçet's Disease
    ベーチェット病
70. Carpal Tunnel Syndrome
    手根管症候群
71. Pseudogout
    偽痛風
72. Vasculitis
    血管炎
73. Cryoglobulinemia
    クリオグロブリン血症
74. Fibromyalgia
    線維筋痛症
75. Gout
    痛風
76. Hypersensitivity Vasculitis
    過敏性血管炎
77. Microscopic Polyangiitis
    顕微鏡的多発動脈炎
78. Osteomyelitis
    骨髄炎
79. Polyarteritis Nodosa
    結節性多発動脈
80. Polymyalgia Rheumatica
    リウマチ性多発筋痛症
81. Psoriatic Arthritis
    乾癬性関節炎
82. Rheumatoid Arthritis
    関節リウマチ
83. Sjögren's Syndrome
    シェーグレン症候群
84. Systemic Lupus Erythematosus
    全身性エリテマトーデス
85. Systemic Sclerosis (Scleroderma)
    全身性強皮症（強皮症）
86. Takayasu's Arteritis
    高安動脈炎
87. Granulomatosis with Polyangiitis (Wegener's)
    ウェゲナー肉芽腫症

METABOLIC DISORDERS　097
代謝性疾患

- *88.* Acromegaly
  先端巨大症
- *89.* Myxedema
  粘液水腫
- *90.* Diabetes Insipidus
  尿崩症
- *91.* Type 1 Diabetes
  1型糖尿病
- *92.* Type 2 Diabetes
  2型糖尿病
- *93.* Diabetic Ketoacidosis
  糖尿病性ケトアシドーシス
- *94.* Cushing's Syndrome
  クッシング症候群
- *95.* Hyperthyroidism
  甲状腺機能亢進症
- *96.* Hypoparathyroidism
  副甲状腺機能低下症
- *97.* Osteoporosis
  骨粗鬆症
- *98.* Panhypopituitarism
  (Sheehan's Syndrome)
  汎下垂機能低下症
  （シーハン症候群）
- *99.* Pheochromocytoma
  褐色細胞腫
- *100.* Addison's Disease
  アジソン病
- *101.* Primary Hyperparathyroidism
  原発性副甲状腺機能亢進症
- *102.* Multinodular Colloid Goiter
  多結節性コロイド甲状腺腫

TOXINS　113
中毒

- *103.* Acetaminophen Poisoning
  アセトアミノフェン中毒
- *104.* Arsenic Poisoning
  ヒ素中毒
- *105.* Digitalis Poisoning
  ジギタリス中毒
- *106.* Cyanide Poisoning
  シアン化合物中毒
- *107.* Isoniazid Poisoning
  イソニアジド中毒
- *108.* Lead Poisoning
  鉛中毒
- *109.* Lithium Poisoning
  リチウム中毒
- *110.* Salicylate Poisoning
  サリチル酸中毒

CONGENITAL 123
先天性疾患

- *111.* Wilson's Disease
  ウイルソン病
- *112.* Acid Maltase Deficiency
  ポンペ病（Pompe Disease）
- *113.* Cor Triatriatum
  三心房心
- *114.* Huntington's Disease
  ハンチントン舞踏病
- *115.* Hemochromatosis
  ヘモクロマトーシス
- *116.* Homocystinemia
  高ホモシスチン血症
- *117.* Protein C and S Deficiencies
  プロテインＣ欠乏症，
  プロテインＳ欠乏症

デザイン：山本　誠（山本誠デザイン室）

VASCULAR DISEASES

血管性疾患

1.

Angina Pectoris
狭心症

Many patients with this condition deny chest pain; instead, they will report heartburn or even abdominal pain.

「多くの狭心症患者は胸痛を否定する．そのかわり，胸やけ，腹痛といった表現すらする」

Visceral pain is much less well localized by the brain, and myocardial ischemia thus may present in a wide variety of ways. It is important to consider the risk factors for similar disease.

内臓痛は大脳によって限局した痛みとして認識されにくい傾向があります＊．このように，心筋虚血はさまざまな訴えとして表現されます．心筋虚血と類似する疾患の危険因子を考慮することが重要です．

［訳者注］
＊大脳は内臓からの疼痛シグナルを，同じ脊髄レベルの後角を経た皮膚からの疼痛シグナルとして認識します．心筋虚血は心筋内の求心性痛覚神経終末を刺激します．この神経線維は交感神経幹を通り，胸髄1～5レベルの左側分節部に入り，心筋虚血はT1～5の体表部の痛みとして自覚されます．痛みのインパルスは，上・下方，右側に伝導するため，頸部（C3），肩（C4），上腹部（T6），右胸部の痛みとして自覚されることがあります．

2.

Aortic Dissection
大動脈解離

Though symptoms are very similar to those of acute myocardial infarction, but the onset is abrupt; myocardial ischemia comes on over a matter of several minutes.

「大動脈解離の症状は心筋梗塞と酷似するが，発症は突然である．心筋虚血は数分かけて症状が起こってくる」

Aortic dissection is an extremely uncommon medical condition, but missing the diagnosis has serious consequences. In dissection, the intimal tear in the aorta occurs suddenly, and the next heart beat forces a column blood into the vessel's media, producing severe pain; the patient is often hypertensive as well.

　大動脈解離はきわめて稀な病態です．しかし，診断を誤ると不幸な転帰が待っています．解離では突然に大動脈内膜に亀裂が生じ，心拍が拍動性血流を血管中膜へ押し出すため，激烈な痛みを生じます．血圧上昇も頻繁に観察されます*．

［訳者注］
*以下のパールも参考にしてください．
In a patient with chest pain who appears to be in shock with an elevated blood pressure, the diagnosis is aortic dissection.
「ショック状態にみえる血圧が高い胸痛患者の診断は大動脈解離である」
　ショックでは皮膚が冷たく蒼白で冷汗を伴います．大動脈解離の患者では，激烈な胸痛がショック様の外観をもたらしますが，高血圧と大動脈解離の関係は，臨床的外観と血圧の不一致を起こします．（『ティアニー先生の診断入門第2版』より）

3.

Aortic Coarctation
大動脈縮窄症

When vascular claudication presents in a young person with hypertension, listen to the back; you may hear the typical murmur of this congenital disorder.

「高血圧を伴った若年者に血管性跛行を認めたら，背部を聴診しなさい．先天性疾患である大動脈縮窄の典型的雑音を聴取するかもしれない」

Aortic coarctation produces reduction in blood flow distal to the left subclavian artery, thus causing reduced perfusion to the kidneys and to the lower extremities. In young people without pre-existing atherosclerosis, it can be a cause of discomfort in the thighs while walking, or even simply a feeling of heaviness when the patient is walking. The characteristic murmur of adult coarctation is best heard in the back.

大動脈縮窄症では左鎖骨下動脈から遠位の血流が低下し，腎・下肢の灌流低下が起こります．アテローム性動脈硬化のない若年者に，歩行時の大腿部の不快感，もしくは単に足が重い感覚を引き起こします．成人の大動脈縮窄症患者の典型的雑音は，背部で最もよく聴取されます．

4.

Aortic Insufficiency
大動脈弁閉鎖不全

In evaluating a diastolic heart murmur, the intensity of the first heart sound may be very helpful; it is an important aortic regurgitation, the first heart sound is often absent.

「拡張期雑音を評価するときは，S_1 の強さが重要かつ大いに参考になる．大動脈弁閉鎖不全では S_1 の欠如が稀ではない」

Because an insufficient aortic valve results in backflow of blood into the left ventricle, the mitral leaflets are nearly closed at the time of ventricular systole; thus, no sound is made by this closure, which ordinarily accounts for the majority of the first heart sound.

大動脈弁閉鎖不全では血液が左室に逆流するため，収縮期への移行時には，僧帽弁尖がほとんど閉鎖しかかっています．これにより，通常，S_1 の大半を占める僧帽弁の閉鎖音がなくなります．

［訳者注］
大動脈弁閉鎖不全をきたす疾患
血管性疾患(Vascular)：長期の高血圧，大動脈解離，大動脈瘤
感染症(Infectious)：感染性心内膜炎，梅毒
腫瘍性疾患(Neoplastic)：粘液腫
自己免疫性疾患(Autoimmune)：リウマチ熱，高安動脈炎，強直性脊椎炎
先天性疾患(Congenital)：二尖弁，マルファン(Marfan)症候群

5.

Aortic Stenosis
大動脈弁狭窄

A loud aortic outflow murmur usually means mild aortic stenosis; the softer the murmur, the worse the stenosis.

「大きな大動脈流出路の雑音は，通常中等度の大動脈弁狭窄を意味する．雑音が弱いと，狭窄が強い」

As the valve becomes increasingly narrowed, the amount of flow through it becomes softer and softer, resulting in a reduction of the loudness of the murmur. Another clue to severity is a very narrow pulse pressure and a delayed carotid upstroke.

弁が狭くなるにつれて，狭窄部を通過する血流は減少し，結果的に雑音の強さが小さくなります．他の重症度を判断する鍵となるものに，脈圧がきわめて小さいこと（小脈），頸動脈の立ち上がりが遅延すること（遅脈）があります．

［訳者注］
大動脈弁狭窄をきたす疾患
自己免疫性疾患（Autoimmune）：リウマチ熱
代謝性疾患（Metabolic）：石灰化（糖尿病による腎不全患者に多い）
変性疾患（Degenerative）：変性性
先天性疾患（Congenital）：二尖弁

6.

Mitral Stenosis
僧帽弁狭窄

Do not forget this diagnosis in a patient with "idiopathic pulmonary hypertension."

「いわゆる特発性肺高血圧症の患者では，僧帽弁狭窄を忘れないこと」

　The rumbling diastolic murmur of mitral stenosis is challenging to hear even in the best of circumstances; however, the inflow obstruction to the left ventricle from the left atrium results in pulmonary hypertension, often quite chronic. Thus, an echocardiogram is essential before the diagnosis of idiopathic pulmonary hypertension is made.

　僧帽弁狭窄の拡張期ランブルは，最良の状況でも聴取するのが困難です．しかし，左房から左室への流入が阻害されると，稀でなく，本当に慢性的な肺高血圧が引き起こされます．したがって，特発性肺高血圧症の診断をくだす前に，心臓超音波が必須なのです．

［訳者注］
僧帽弁狭窄をきたす疾患
自己免疫性疾患（Autoimmune）：リウマチ熱，全身性エリテマトーデス〔リブマン・サックス（Libman-Sacks）心内膜炎による〕
変性疾患（Degenerative）：僧帽弁輪石灰化
先天性疾患（Congenital）：先天性僧帽弁狭窄

7.

Mitral Regurgitation
僧帽弁閉鎖不全

Do not overlook the carotid pulse in assessing systolic murmur; mitral regurgitation typically causes a rapid up-and-down quality to this pulse.

「収縮期雑音の評価で頸動脈拍動を見落としてはならない．僧帽弁閉鎖不全は典型的に立ち上がりの速い反跳脈を引き起こす」

Because the left ventricle empties rapidly when the mitral valve is insufficient, the pulse in the neck is what can be considered an up-and-down pulse, with the same general morphology as that of aortic insufficiency. More importantly, because it is a systolic murmur, the contrast between mitral regurgitation and aortic stenosis can often be made just by the quality of the neck pulse.

　僧帽弁閉鎖不全では左室の収縮が急速に終了するため，頸動脈拍動が大動脈弁閉鎖不全と同じ性質をもつ反跳脈となります．さらに重要なのは，同じ収縮期雑音を示す僧帽弁閉鎖不全と大動脈弁狭窄のコントラストが，頸動脈拍動の性質（反跳脈と小脈・遅脈）によって頻繁に明らかにされることです．

［訳者注］
僧帽弁閉鎖不全をきたす疾患
血管性疾患（Vascular）：乳頭筋断裂（心筋梗塞による）
感染症（Infectious）：感染性心内膜炎
腫瘍性疾患（Neoplastic）：粘液腫
自己免疫性疾患（Autoimmune）：リウマチ熱，全身性エリテマトーデス（リブマン・サックス心内膜炎による）
変性疾患（Degenerative）：僧帽弁輪石灰化
先天性疾患（Congenital）：先天性僧帽弁閉鎖不全
特発性疾患（Idiopathic）：拡張型心筋症，腱索断裂

8.

Atrial Fibrillation
心房細動

Direct thrombin inhibitors such as dabigatran are the wave of the future in preventing embolic events in patients with this rhythm.

「ダビガトランのような直接トロンビン阻害剤は心房細動患者の塞栓予防の将来の波になる」

Studies have shown that the direct thrombin inhibitor dabigatran is superior to warfarin in the prevention of stroke in atrial fibrillation, and will likely be approved for other uses as well; it has a particular value in that it does not require monitoring the prothrombin time, but cannot be used in renal insufficiency.

いくつかの研究において，直接トロンビン阻害剤ダビガトランがワルファリンよりも心房細動の脳塞栓予防に優れているという結果が示されました．さらに，他の病態への応用も同様に認可されるでしょう．プロトロンビン時間をモニターする必要がないのが大きな利点です．しかし，腎不全患者に使うことができません．

9.

Atrial Flutter
心房粗動

If a patient with COPD has a heart rate which is 140–150 and regular, the diagnosis is atrial flutter.

「COPD 患者が 140〜150/分・整の頻脈を示したら，診断は心房粗動である」

In patients with chronic pulmonary disease, atrial arrhythmias are common, with atrial flutter and multifocal atrial tachycardia being the most common. Atrial flutter can be separated from MAT because it is regular, and because the rate of 150 indicates a 2：1 AV block, which, on occasion, may be difficult to see on the surface electrocardiogram, but is considerably faster than would be appropriate for the patient's level of activity.

慢性肺疾患の患者において，心房性不整脈は珍しくありません．心房粗動，多源性心房頻拍が最も代表的なものです．心房粗動と多源性心房頻拍は，以下の点から鑑別できるでしょう．心房粗動は整脈を示し，心拍数 150 は心電図上で見分けるのが困難な 2：1 の房室ブロックを意味し，患者の活動度にふさわしい心拍よりも，かなり速い心拍数を示します*．

［訳者注］
＊多源性心房頻拍の心房，心室のレートは通常 100〜150/分です．

10.

Atrial Septal Defect
心房中隔欠損症

Ninety-five percent (95%) of adults with this congenital defect have a right ventricular conduction disturbance.

「成人心房中隔欠損症の患者の 95％に右室の伝導障害がある」

ASD is likely the most common congenital cardiac abnormality encountered in adulthood. The right ventricular conduction disturbance may result from the left-to-right interatrial shunt, increasing the workload of the right ventricle. Also commonly encountered in fixed splitting is wide, fixed splitting of the second heart sound.

心房中隔欠損症は成人でみつかる先天性心疾患のなかで最も多いものです．右室の伝導障害は，左-右シャントによる右室の仕事量の増加に由来すると考えられます．S_2 は固定性分裂で幅広く分裂します．

［訳者注］
　S_2 の幅広い分裂（$A_2 \rightarrow P_2$ の順に分裂，吸気時により明瞭）では，右室の収縮完了が遅れています．鑑別には，完全右脚ブロック，肺高血圧症，肺動脈弁狭窄，重篤な僧帽弁閉鎖不全（左室の収縮が逆流のため早期に完了する）があります．S_2 の奇異性分裂（吸気よりも呼気時に分裂が明瞭，$P_2 \rightarrow A_2$ の順に分裂）では，左室の収縮完了が遅れています．鑑別には，完全左脚ブロック，重度の大動脈弁狭窄があります．ASD では左-右シャントのため，呼吸とは関係なく固定した分裂（$A_2 \rightarrow P_2$ の順に分裂）を示します．

11.

Congestive Heart Failure
うっ血性心不全

Ninety percent (90%) of congestive heart failure in adults is caused by either ischemic, hypertensive, or valvular heart disease, in that order; the most important to consider on a first visit is the latter.

「成人のうっ血性心不全の90%は,虚血性,高血圧性,もしくは心臓弁膜症によって引き起こされる.この順番で最も重要なのは心臓弁膜症を最初に検討することである」

Ischemic and hypertensive heart disease, though commonest in most societies, are treated more or less identically. On the other hand, valvular heart disease is with few exceptions a mechanical problem, requiring a mechanical, or in this case surgical, solution. Thus, all patients presenting for the first time with symptoms and signs of heart failure should have a cardiac echo as part of the early assessment, to exclude a completely curable disorder such as aortic stenosis.

虚血性,高血圧性心疾患は,あらゆる社会で最も多いものですが,多かれ少なかれ同じような治療が行われています.一方,心臓弁膜症は2〜3の例外はあるものの,機械的な問題であり,機械的,もしくは外科的な治療を必要とします.したがって,うっ血性心不全の最初の症状・徴候を認めたすべての患者において,大動脈弁狭窄のような完全に治せる疾患を除外するために,早期の評価として心臓超音波が行われなくてはなりません.

12.

Constrictive Pericarditis
収縮性心膜炎

This surgically treatable disorder is the most commonly misdiagnosed cause of new-onset ascites.

「この外科的に治療しうる疾患は新たに発生した腹水の原因として最も誤診される」

　Most patients with this condition come to the physician with what appears to be either heart failure, given elevated neck veins and edema. Any cause of pericarditis, however, may ultimately result in scarring, impairing the filling of the heart from the great vessels. The pressure is appreciably high so that ascites is typically present on first visit and this is seldom the case in congestive heart failure. This is yet another reason why echocardiography should be performed on all patients with suspected heart failure.

　収縮性心膜炎患者のほとんどは，心不全様徴候，高い頸静脈波，浮腫を呈して医師のもとを訪れます．心膜炎の原因が何であれ，最終的には瘢痕化をきたし，大静脈から心臓への血液還流が阻害されます．明らかに圧が高く，典型的には初診時に腹水を認めます．これはうっ血性心不全ではありません．これが心不全を疑うすべての患者で，心臓超音波を行うもう１つのさらなる理由なのです．

13.

Hypertension
高血圧症

One can screen for secondary causes easily in the office; all pheochromocytomas have an orthostatic fall in blood pressure, and the typical patient with hyperaldosteronism has a serum sodium greater than 140 and a urine potassium over 40.

「二次性高血圧のスクリーニングは外来で簡単にできる．すべての褐色細胞腫患者に起立性の血圧低下を認め，典型的な高アルドステロン症患者では血清ナトリウム 140 mEq/L 以上，尿中カリウム 40 mEq/L 以上である」

The vast majority of patients with elevated blood pressure have no reversible cause of this condition, and are simply treated without assessment. Because patients with pheochromocytoma have chronic vasoconstriction, their blood pressure will fall upon standing because of the hypovolemia. Likewise, the effect of excessive mineralocorticoid results in elevated serum sodium and an elevated urinary potassium. Both of these are inexpensive, and should be done on a first visit for elevated blood pressure. Many patients with this condition make the diagnosis themselves by measuring their blood pressure in a pharmacy.

血圧の上昇した大多数の患者では，可逆的な原因は存在せず，単に評価なく治療されています．褐色細胞腫患者では慢性的な血管収縮のため，循環血液量減少による起立時の血圧低下が起こります．同様に，鉱質コルチコイド過剰の影響は，血清ナトリウムを上昇させ，尿中カリウム排泄を増加させます．どちらも費用がかからないので，血圧上昇のために初めて受診した患者で評価してください．高血圧症患者の多くは，薬局で自分の血圧を測定し，自ら高血圧症の診断を行っています．

14.
Ventricular Tachycardia
心室頻拍

Listen carefully to the heart in a patient with wide complex tachycardia: varying intensity of S_1 may tell you that it is VT.

「QRS幅の広い頻拍患者の聴診は注意深く行いなさい．強さが変化する S_1 は心室頻拍の存在を示唆する」

In ventricular tachycardia, atrioventricular dissociation is present, but may be difficult to appreciate on cardiograms. The result is differing length of PR intervals, which causes the first heart sound to vary in its loudness. Auscultation is always important in assessing a tachyarrhythmia.

心室頻拍では房室解離が存在します．しかし，心電図で認識するのは困難でしょう．PR間隔が異なるため，S_1 の強さが変化します．聴診は頻拍性不整脈の評価で常に重要なのです．

INFECTIOUS DISEASES

感染症

15.

Brucellosis
ブルセラ症

Brucellosis. A popularly considered diagnosis in unexplained fever, but the correct epidemiology must be present for it to be considered seriously.

「ブルセラ症．説明のつかない発熱において一般に考慮される．しかし，ブルセラ症を強く疑うには正確な疫学が存在する」

Brucellosis is a chronic febrile disease characterized by low back pain, and with virtually no exceptions, an occupational history of working as a veterinarian or in a slaughterhouse; likewise, ingestion of unpasteurized milk or cheese may cause this, from a different *Brucella* species. Because of the nonspecific nature of many of the clinical findings, it then becomes important to obtain an occupational and dietary history because of the clinical similarity to lymphoma, endocarditis, and tuberculosis.

ブルセラ症は腰痛を特徴とする慢性的な発熱疾患です．例外なく，獣医，屠畜場での職業歴，同様に，殺菌されていない牛乳やチーズの摂取歴が，異なるブルセラ菌種によるブルセラ症を引き起こします．非特異的な多くの症状を呈し，リンパ腫，感染性心内膜炎，結核と類似するため，職業歴・食事歴の聴取がとても重要なのです．

16.

Cat Scratch Disease
ネコひっかき病

This need not be transmitted by scratch; even licking or a bite may do the job.

「ひっかきによる感染だけでなく，なめられても咬まれても感染する」

Affected animals, which are usually kittens obtained from an animal shelter, have strongly positive blood cultures for *Bartonella henselae*, and thus are highly contagious. Interestingly, the cats themselves show no sign of sickness. The same organism causes bacillary angiomatosis in HIV-AIDS patients.

感染した動物は，主にアニマルシェルターにいる子ネコです．*Bartonella henselae* が血液培養において陽性で，感染性が強いのです．興味深いことに，ネコそのものは病的症状を示しません．同じものが HIV-AIDS 患者の細菌性血管腫症を引き起こします．

17.

Cholera
コレラ

A condition characterized by extremely high volume, watery diarrhea, which can be lethal due to hemoconcentration and venous thrombosis.

「大量の水様性下痢により特徴づけられる病態は，血液濃縮・静脈血栓のため死に至ることがある」

Although the causative organism, *Vibrio cholerae*, is not especially invasive, it, in essence, paralyzes the ability of the small intestine to reabsorb fluid, creating an extreme diarrheal illness. The key to survival is rapid replacement of fluids, and inhibitors of cAMP such as cola may also be of some value. There has been a recent epidemic of this in the country of Haiti.

コレラの原因菌である *Vibrio cholerae* は，さほど侵襲的ではありません．しかし，本質的に小腸の水分再吸収能力を麻痺させ，大量の下痢を引き起こします*．生存のための鍵は急速な輸液です．また，コーラのような cAMP 阻害薬も効果的でしょう．最近，ハイチでの流行がありました[1,2]．

［訳者注］
＊コレラ毒素は腸管上皮細胞の cAMP のレベルを高めます．cAMP は絨毛細胞でのナトリウム吸収を阻害し，陰窩細胞ではクロールの分泌を活発化させます．結果的に腸管内の塩化ナトリウム濃度が上昇し，下痢が起こります．

［文献］
1) Walton DA, Ivers LC. Responding to Cholera in Post-Earthquake Haiti. N Engl J Med 364: 3-5, 2011.
2) Chin C-S, et al. The Origin of the Haitian Cholera Outbreak Strain. N Engl J Med 364: 33-42, 2011.

18. Typhoid Fever
腸チフス

Look for leukopenia and bradycardia; if an increased heart rate and elevated white count develop, the patient has perforated the ileum.

「白血球減少・徐脈を探しなさい．もし頻脈・白血球増多を認めたら，患者は回腸穿孔を起こしている」

Like many *salmonella* infections, typhoid has a heart rate slower than the clinician expects given the height of the fever, and likewise, a white blood count less than expected given how ill the patient is. Because the distal ileum is commonly affected by the organism, it has a tendency to rupture, causing superinfection by other organisms, and thus a change in the white count and heart rate. The clinician should also be on the alert for faint, pink macules on the trunk, which are called "rose spots."

他のサルモネラ感染症と同じように，腸チフスでは医師が発熱から予想するよりも心拍は遅く*，同様に，白血球数は重症度から予想するよりも少ないのです．遠位回腸は病原菌に侵されやすく，穿孔することがあり，他の細菌のさらなる感染を引き起こし，白血球数，心拍数が変化します．体幹の淡いピンク色の斑である「バラ疹」にも注意してください．

［訳者注］
*比較的徐脈をきたす疾患
感染症（Infectious）：腸チフス，クラミジア，レジオネラ，ブルセラ症，黄熱
腫瘍性疾患（Neoplastic）：リンパ腫
医原性の修飾（発熱があっても脈を速くできない状態）：β遮断薬の内服，ペースメーカー挿入

The Best Clinical Pearls of Dr.Tierney

19.

Leprosy
ハンセン病

The causative organism of leprosy (Mycobacterium leprae) can only be grown in the feet of armadillos, a small ectotherm seen along roads in the Deep South of America.

「ハンセン病の病原体である *Mycobacterium leprae* は，南米奥地の道に沿ってみられる小型外温動物であるアルマジロの足でのみ培養できる」

It is uncertain as to how it was discovered that this was the only way it was possible to culture this organism, which can have so many different clinical manifestations. It may be that the bacteria favors relatively cool environments, and the feet of any organism ordinarily have lower core temperatures than other parts of the body.

多彩な症状を呈しうるこの細菌を培養する方法は，アルマジロの足でのみ可能ですが*，どのようにして発見されたのか，実はわかっていません．おそらく，細菌は比較的低温の環境を好み，どんな生物でも，足は他の体のどの部位よりも中心温が低いからでしょう．

［訳者注］
*科学が進歩した今日でも *Mycobacterium leprae* は，人工培地，組織培養細胞を用いた培養ができない菌です．

20.

Leptospirosis
レプトスピラ症

Jaundice and red eyes in a person living near water is leptospirosis until proven otherwise.

「黄疸と赤い眼を呈し水辺近くに住む患者では他の診断がつくまでレプトスピラ症を考えなさい」

Leptospiras are excreted in the urine of rats, and in consequence, find their way into water, especially stagnant water which is intermediate between salt and fresh water. Occasional patients also have aseptic meningitis, and muscle pain with elevated CK levels may be found as well in this elusive condition.

レプトスピラはネズミの尿に排泄され，結果的に海水と真水の中間くらいの汽水域のよどんだ水の中へ混入します．ときに，患者は無菌性髄膜炎も呈し，とらえどころのないこの疾患では，CK 上昇を伴う筋痛を認めることもあります．

21.

The Best Clinical Pearls of Dr.Tierney

Bacterial Meningitis
細菌性髄膜炎

In a patient with headache, stiff neck, and fever without focal neurological signs, do the lumbar puncture first: obtaining a CT is a waste of valuable time.

「頭痛・項部硬直・発熱を呈し神経学的巣症状のない患者では，腰椎穿刺をまず行う．CTは貴重な時間の浪費である」

Because of the widespread availability of CT and MR scanning, many clinicians routinely obtain these studies in patients who ultimately turn out to have meningitis. There is no evidence that performing a spinal tap first in patients without focal neurological deficits results in herniation of the brainstem, and obtaining the imaging studies consumes time which is crucial to the outcome of this serious infection. *Pneumococcus, Meningococcus, and Hemophilus* (in children) account for 90% of cases.

　CTとMRIが広く利用できるようになり，多くの医師は最終的に細菌性髄膜炎と診断される患者において，これらの画像を決まったこととしてオーダーしています．神経学的巣症状のない患者に，まず腰椎穿刺を行うことが脳幹部のヘルニアを起こすというエビデンスはありません．画像を撮ることは，この重篤な疾患の帰結にとって決定的な時間を浪費することになります．肺炎球菌，髄膜炎菌，ヘモフィルス（小児）が細菌性髄膜炎の90％を占めます．

22.

Pertussis
百日咳

This re-emerging disease is the cause of the highest benign white counts in medicine.

「この再興した疾患は，医学における最も著明かつ良性の白血球増多の原因である」

Because of the recent anti-vaccination movement in the United States, and of under-vaccination elsewhere in the world, this disorder is becoming more common. It is the cause of classic whooping cough in children, in whom it may be life-threatening, and in whom extraordinary elevations of white blood cells are found. In adults, this is ordinarily not seen, and the condition resembles an acute upper respiratory tract infection.

最近の米国における反ワクチン接種の動きや，他のワクチン接種の足りない国々のため，百日咳は著増しています．小児では生命を脅かす古典的咳発作の原因となり，驚くほどの白血球増多を認めます．通常，成人ではこの現象は認められず，急性の上気道感染に似ます．

23.
Pneumococcal Infections
肺炎球菌感染症

Severe chest pain with a shaking chill? Blood cultures will show you pneumococcus tomorrow.

「悪寒戦慄を伴ったひどい胸痛？　明日，血液培養は肺炎球菌陽性を示す」

　Early symptoms typically include pleuritic chest pain, often severe enough to imitate other causes of thoracic discomfort, including myocardial infarction; most patients with pneumonia of other types do not have pleuritic chest pain, especially during the early days of the infection.

　肺炎球菌肺炎の初期の症状には，心筋梗塞を含む胸部不快感を呈する疾患に類似する，きわめて強い胸膜性胸痛が典型的に含まれます．肺炎球菌以外の肺炎患者の多くは，特に感染初期には胸膜性胸痛を示しません．

24.
Streptococcal Pharyngitis
連鎖球菌咽頭炎

Despite the serious nature of pharyngeal diphtheria, fever is higher in Strep throat.

「咽頭ジフテリアの重篤な経過にもかかわらず，発熱は連鎖球菌咽頭炎で高い」

Ordinarily, clinicians seeing an especially inflamed pharynx consider diphtheria, mononucleosis, and *streptococcal* infections on their diagnostic list; however, if the body temperature is above 39 degrees C, diphtheria is likely not to be the diagnosis, as it rarely causes more than a low-grade elevation in temperature.

通常，医師は咽頭に炎症を認めると，ジフテリア，伝染性単核球症，連鎖球菌感染を鑑別診断として考えるでしょう．しかし，体温が39℃以上なら，ジフテリアらしくありません．ジフテリアでは高熱が稀にしか起こりません．

25. Primary Syphilis
第1期梅毒

A painless genital or oral ulcer should be considered to be syphilis until proven otherwise, irrespective of the sexual history.

「無痛性の陰部もしくは口腔内潰瘍では，性交歴と関係なく他の診断がつくまで梅毒を考えなさい」

Although there are numerous causes of oral and genital ulcers, syphilis has a very specific form of treatment in penicillin, and is notoriously difficult to obtain a sexual history in many cases; in primary syphilis the RPR is only positive in 60% of patients.

口腔内潰瘍と陰部潰瘍を引き起こす原因はいくつもありますが，梅毒にはペニシリン投与という特異的な治療があります．また，性交歴を得るのは，多くの例でおそろしく困難です．第1期梅毒ではRPR（rapid plasma reagin）が60％しか陽性になりません．

26.

Secondary Syphilis
第 2 期梅毒

Any rash involving the palms and soles should be considered secondary syphilis until proven otherwise.

「手掌・足底のどんな皮疹も他の診断がつくまで第 2 期梅毒を考えなさい*¹」

Again, similar to primary syphilis, the sexual contact history may be very difficult to obtain; however, the RPR is 100% sensitive. Be careful of a Herxheimer reaction shortly after the first dose of penicillin, this being a transient shock-like state due to lysis of the spirochetes; the skin lesions typically become temporarily exaggerated.

再度強調しますが，第 1 期梅毒と同様に性交歴を聴取するのは，とても難しいことです．しかし，RPR は感度 100％です．最初のペニシリン投与後のヘルクスハイマー（Herxheimer）反応に注意してください．これは一過性のショック様の状態で，スピロヘータの溶解が原因です*²．典型例では一時的に皮疹が悪化します．

［訳者注］
*¹ 第 2 期梅毒の播種性丘疹落屑型発疹のことです．過角化を示します．上腕内側上顆のリンパ節腫脹を伴うことがあります．
*² スピロヘータの溶解によって生じるリポ蛋白の放出がヘルクスハイマー反応を引き起こすと考えられています．

27. Tuberculosis
結核

In HIV-infected patients, if the clinical picture looks like tuberculosis, it's not, and if it doesn't, it is.

「HIV患者では臨床像が結核にみえても結核でなく，結核にみえなくても結核のことがある」

In patients infected with HIV, tuberculosis is a particularly common infection, but unlike reactivation tuberculosis, it tends to occur in a primary pattern, as an infiltrate with regional hilar adenopathy in the mid-lung field; apical cavities, typical of reactivation tuberculosis in immunologically normal persons, are more apt to be emphysema or a saprophytic infection which need not be treated.

結核はHIV患者において頻繁に経験されます．しかし，結核の再活性化と異なり，局所的な肺門リンパ節腫脹を伴う中肺野の浸潤影のような初感染パターンとして起こる傾向があります．典型的な免疫正常患者の再活性化で認められる肺尖部の空洞化は，肺気腫，もしくは治療の必要のない腐性の感染を引き起こします．

28.

Coccidiomycosis
コクシジオイデス症

If a patient with any febrile condition has recently been driving in California's Central Valley, this fungal disorder should be high on the list of conditions considered by clinicians.

「発熱を有するどんな患者も最近カリフォルニア中部渓谷にドライブしたなら，この真菌感染が鑑別の上位に入る」

The dry, desert-like weather conditions of the western United States, including California, New Mexico, and Arizona are an ideal culture medium to produce the highly infectious arthrospores of this disorder; the degree of infectivity is so high that only a brief drive through endemic areas on a windy day in late summer is enough to cause an illness usually characterized by a pulmonary infiltrate and arthralgias.

カリフォルニア，ニューメキシコ，アリゾナを含むアメリカ西部の乾燥した砂漠のような気候は，感染性の高いこの感染症の分節型分生子の理想的な培地です．風の吹く夏の終わり頃に，流行地域を短時間ドライブしただけでも，通常，肺の浸潤影と関節痛によって特徴づけられるこの感染症を引き起こすのに十分であり，感染性はきわめて高いのです．

29.

Cryptococcosis
クリプトコッカス症

During the early years of the HIV-AIDS epidemic, this was the most common form of meningitis admitted to U. S. hospitals.

「HIV-AIDS の流行初期の間，クリプトコッカス症は米国の入院髄膜炎において最も多いタイプであった」

While cryptococcosis had formerly been observed only rarely in training hospitals in America and elsewhere, being noted only in patients with Hodgkin's disease and those receiving anti-cancer medications, it occurred in nearly epidemic proportions in people with impaired host defensive mechanisms because of the HIV virus; 95% of these patients have positive serum *cryptococcal* antigen.

以前，クリプトコッカス症は，米国やその他の国の研修病院において稀にしか認められませんでした．ホジキン病や抗腫瘍薬を投与されているような患者にしか認められなかったのです．しかし，HIV による宿主の免疫能が低下した患者において，流行といえるほどの割合で認められました．これらの HIV 患者の 95％で血清クリプトコッカス抗原が陽性です．

30.

Histoplasmosis
ヒストプラズマ症

In Americans whose Social Security number begins with 2, 3, or 4, and who have calcifications on their chest x-ray, this is the diagnosis.

「米国人で社会保障番号が 2 か 3 か 4 で始まり，胸部 X 線写真上石灰化陰影を認めたら，診断はヒストプラズマ症である」

Social Security numbers in the U. S. are distributed according to the geographical location of where the individual received their card; those with SSNs starting with 2, 3, or 4 are spread across the great river valleys of North America, a highly endemic area for histoplasmosis. Patients with normal immune systems develop disseminated disease in 1 : 250, 000; in persons with HIV-AIDS it is considerably more common as a systemic, typhoidal illness.

米国の社会保障番号は，個人が受け取るカードの地理的な位置で分類されています．2，3，4 で始まる地域は，北米の大渓谷を横断するように分布し，ヒストプラズマ症の濃厚な流行地域なのです．免疫能正常者では播種性ヒストプラズマ症の発症率が 25 万人に 1 人です．HIV-AIDS 患者ではその頻度が高く，チフス性の症状を呈します．

31.

Pneumocystis Pneumonia (PCP)
ニューモシスチス肺炎

Do not be afraid to use steroids during the early treatment of severe cases; there is often a Herxheimer-like effect worsening the condition if you do not.

「ニューモシスチス肺炎重症例の初期治療においてステロイド投与をおそれなくてよい．投与しないとヘルクスハイマー様反応*で状態が悪化する」

It was noticed early in the HIV-AIDS epidemic that patients with relatively serious infection tended to worsen their pulmonary status, often requiring intubation, shortly after antibiotic treatment was begun. This appears to be due to a local inflammatory reaction to the killing of the fungus, and prophylactic use of high-dose of steroids may prevent this; it is not intuitive given that this infection occurs entirely in already immunosuppressed patients.

　HIV-AIDS の流行初期に観察されたのは，比較的重症のニューモシスチス肺炎患者の肺の状態が，抗菌薬投与後間もなく，気管内挿管を必要とするような悪化傾向を示したことでした．これは真菌の死滅に対する局所の炎症反応に由来するようです．予防的な高用量のステロイド投与がこれを防止します．ニューモシスチス肺炎が既に免疫不全に陥っている患者に起こるため，ステロイドは直感的に投与されるものではありませんね．

［訳者注］
＊パール 26「第 2 期梅毒」(29 頁) を参照してください．

32.
Cysticercosis
嚢虫症

The most common cause of seizures in young adults in Central America.

「中米の若年者のてんかん発作の原因として最も多いのは嚢虫症である」

The causative larva of *T. solium* favors location in the central nervous system, where it may cause seizures; in addition, it is one of the few causes of eosinophilic meningitis, and imaging studies show intracerebral calcification of cysts.

嚢虫症の原因である *Taenia solium** の幼虫は，てんかん発作を起こしうる中枢神経を好みます．さらに，好酸球性髄膜炎を起こす数少ない原因の1つです．画像では脳内の嚢胞石灰化を示します．

［訳者注］
* *Taenia solium* は有鉤条虫です．

33.

Schistosomiasis
ヒト住血吸虫症

In patients who have lived in the endemic area, even years earlier, investigate this possibility before diagnosing pulmonary hypertension due to other causes.

「流行地域に住んでいた患者ではそれが何年も前でも，他の原因による肺高血圧症と診断する前にヒト住血吸虫症の可能性を考慮しなさい」

　In schistosomiasis, the causative parasite lives for decades in the intestine, continuing to lay eggs, which upon entering the portal system produce pre-sinusoidal fibrosis and porto-systemic collateral blood flow. The eggs thus bypass the liver, end up in the small vessels of the lung, causing pulmonary hypertension. Unlike strongyloidiasis, there is no eosinophilia present in the chronic form of this disease.

　ヒト住血吸虫症では原因となる寄生虫が産卵しつつ，数十年もの間，腸に住み着いています．虫卵は門脈に侵入し，肝類洞前の線維化を引き起こし，門脈-体循環の側副血行を発達させます．したがって，虫卵は肝臓をバイパスし，最終的に肺の小血管に至り，肺高血圧症の原因となります．糞線虫症と異なり，慢性に経過したヒト住血吸虫症でも，好酸球増多は認められません．

［訳者注］
　ヒト住血吸虫症は，*Schistosoma mansoni*, *S. japonicum*, *S. mekongi*, *S. intercalatum*, *S. haematobium* の5種類によって起こります．

34.

Strongyloidiasis
糞線虫症

If the location is right, duodenal ulcer with eosinophilia is strongyloidiasis until proven otherwise.

「流行地域ならば，好酸球増多を伴った十二指腸潰瘍では他の診断がつくまで糞線虫症を考えなさい」

Since the organism resides in the upper part of the small intestine, it may appear to be an acid-peptic lesion on various imaging studies, suggesting complicated ulcer disease; ordinarily, duodenal ulcer is not associated with eosinophilia, and when present, particularly in patients in endemic areas, this diagnosis should be considered in the differential.

糞線虫は上部小腸に寄生するので，いくつかの画像診断では，酸-消化性の複雑な潰瘍病変を示唆するように見えるかもしれません．通常，十二指腸潰瘍は好酸球増多を伴わず，特に，流行地域の患者において好酸球増多を伴った十二指腸潰瘍を認めたら，糞線虫症を鑑別診断として挙げてください．

35.

Fish Tapeworm
広節裂頭条虫

In vitamin B_{12} deficiency in societies where raw fish is a dietary staple, this is your diagnosis.

「おもに生魚を食する地域のビタミン B_{12} 欠乏は，広節裂頭条虫が診断である」

The causative helminth, *Diphyllobothrium latum* may grow to great lengths, even 10 meters or more, in the intestine, and upon occasion, a patient will pass the tapeworm and show it to the physician!; the B_{12} deficiency is due to competition for dietary B_{12} between the host and the parasite.

原因となる条虫，広節裂頭条虫（*Diphyllobothrium latum*）は，消化管で大きく成長し，10 m 以上にも大きくなります．ときに，患者が広節裂頭条虫を排泄し，なんと，それを医師に見せてくれることがあります！　ビタミン B_{12} 欠乏は宿主と寄生虫間のビタミン B_{12} 吸収の競合によって起こります．

The Best Clinical Pearls of Dr.Tierney

36.

Amoebiasis
アメーバ症

Exclude amoebic colitis before administration of steroids for "inflammatory bowel disease"; it is more endemic in many areas than you think.

「いわゆる炎症性腸疾患へのステロイド投与を開始する前にアメーバ性大腸炎を除外しなさい．想像以上に多くの地域で流行している」

Because amoebic colitis can resemble ulcerative colitis both in endoscopic appearance and in clinical presentation, it is essential to exclude it before administration of glucocorticoids, which cause the disease to become systemic. Another form of the disease, amoeboma, can completely mimic carcinoma of the cecum or sigmoid colon.

アメーバ性大腸炎は内視鏡・臨床像が潰瘍性大腸炎に似ているため，アメーバ性大腸炎の全身への拡大を招く糖質コルチコイドの投与前に，アメーバ性大腸炎を除外しなくてはなりません．アメーバ症の他の症状にアメーバ性肉芽腫があります．これは盲腸・Ｓ状結腸癌に酷似します．

37.

Trypanosomiasis (Chagas' Disease)
トリパノソーマ症

The commonest cause of congestive heart failure in South and Central America.

「南米・中米において,うっ血性心不全の最も多い原因はトリパノソーマ症である」

Although often asymptomatic, the parasites may infiltrate the cardiac muscle, as well as the esophagus, causing right-sided congestive heart failure and megaesophagus. Thus, particularly in residents of far southern North America, as well as South and Central America, if no other cause of heart failure evident, think of this condition.

多くは無症状ですが,この寄生虫(*Trypanosoma cruzi*)は,心筋,同様に食道に侵入することがあり,右心不全,巨大食道を引き起こします.このように,特に,北米南部,同様に南米・中米の住民で心不全を起こす他の原因が明らかでないときは,トリパノソーマ症を考慮してください.

38. Visceral Leishmaniasis
内臓型リーシュマニア症

One of the few causes of twice-daily fever spikes in medicine.

「内臓型リーシュマニア症は，1日2回のスパイク状の発熱をきたす医学における数少ない原因の1つである」

For reasons which are unclear, the fever spikes in this disease occur both in the morning and in the evening; only Stills' disease and gonococcal endocarditis produce similar patterns. It is also the cause of the largest spleens encountered in clinical medicine, and more is apt to be seen in soldiers returning from Gulf wars, given the endemicity of this disease there.

理由はわかっていませんが，内臓型リーシュマニア症の発熱は，朝と夕方の2回，スパイク状を呈します．成人スティル病，淋菌性心内膜炎のみが同じパターンを示します．また，内臓型リーシュマニア症は臨床上遭遇する最大の脾腫を呈する疾患です．流行地域で行われた湾岸戦争から帰還した兵士によく認められました．

［訳者注］
リーシュマニア原虫はサシチョウバエ（phlebotomine sandfly）によって媒介されます．

39. Q Fever
Q 熱

The only rickettsial disease without a rash.

「Q 熱は発疹のない唯一のリケッチア症である」

The Q in the name of this disorder does not stand for Queensland, as many believe, but rather, for query, given that, because of the absence of a skin rash, it may present as an elusive febrile illness with granulomatous hepatitis, interstitial pneumonitis, and culture-negative endocarditis.

Q 熱の「Q」は，多くの人が信じるクィーンズランド（Queensland）の略語ではありません．むしろ，発疹がなく，肉芽腫性肝炎，間質性肺炎，血液培養陰性の心内膜炎を伴う，とらえどころのない発熱性疾患であることへの疑問（query）に由来するようです．

［訳者注］
Q 熱は *Coxiella burnetii* 感染によって起こります．

40.

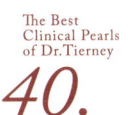

Tsutsugamushi Disease
ツツガムシ病

The characteristic eschar at the site of mite bite may be hidden in the hair on the scalp, and drain to a lymph node behind the ear, making the diagnosis tricky.

「ツツガムシの刺し口の特徴的な血痂が髪に隠れる頭皮にあって，耳介後部のリンパ節が腫脹した場合は，診断が難しい」

Usually the eschar is easily seen, and in fact is often the reason patients seek medical attention. However, if in areas on the body where it may be hidden, and draining to regional lymph nodes commonly not examined by clinicians, it may test one's diagnostic skills.

通常，血痂は簡単に観察できます．実際に，患者は血痂を理由に病院を訪れます．しかし，血痂が体の隠れる部分にあると，所属リンパ節は医師によって触診されません．医師の身体診察能力が試されます．

［訳者注］
　ツツガムシ病の病原体は，*Orientia tsutsugamushi* です．

Cytomegalovirus Disease
サイトメガロウイルス感染症

Think CMV in "mononucleosis" absent a sore throat.

「咽頭炎のないいわゆる単核球症ではサイトメガロウイルス（CMV）感染症を考えなさい」

CMV was once felt to be a consequence of cardiac surgery, and in fact was known as post-pump perfusion syndrome, given fever, systemic symptoms, and organomegaly which occurred several weeks after open heart surgery. It turned out that this was due to this virus contaminating blood transfusions, which are now all tested for this disorder before being administered to patients. There are many clinical manifestations of this condition, especially the retinitis, especially in specifically or non-specifically immunosuppressed patients.

サイトメガロウイルス感染症は，かつて人工心肺後症候群として知られ，心臓手術の結果起こるものと思われていました．開心術後，数週間して，発熱，全身症状，臓器腫大が認められました．今では輸血前にすべて検査されますが，これはサイトメガロウイルスを含んだ血液の輸血が原因だったと判明したのです．サイトメガロウイルス感染症には多くの症状があります．特異的，非特異的であれ，免疫不全の患者では，サイトメガロウイルス網膜炎が起こります．

42.
HIV Infection
HIV 感染症

One of the great success stories in the developed world, but still a tragic cause of enormous mortality around most of the globe.

「先進国の大きな成功の 1 つに HIV 感染症がある．しかし，それは地球のいたるところでいまだ多数の死亡をもたらす悲劇である」

Although unknown prior to 1980, HIV-AIDS became a worldwide global pandemic with millions of deaths annually. There are now more than 20 antiretrovirals which can reconstitute lost immunity, and dramatically extend life expectancy; tragically, most of these are not available in the developing world because of cost and access issues.

1980 年以前に HIV-AIDS は知られていませんでしたが，HIV-AIDS は年間何百万人もの患者が亡くなる世界的流行をきたしました．今や，失われた免疫を再構築できる 20 以上の抗レトロウイルス薬があり，劇的な生存期間の延長が可能となりました．しかし，悲しいことに発展途上国では，費用とアクセスの問題からこれらの薬剤が利用されていません．

43.

Multiple Sclerosis
多発性硬化症

If you diagnose multiple sclerosis over age 50, diagnose something else.

「50歳以上の患者で多発性硬化症を診断したら，真の診断はほかにある」

The onset of multiple sclerosis is nearly always in younger people; the pearl refers to a new diagnosis, as some patients with younger age of onset still have the condition as they pass 50 years of age. In addition, after the age of 50, there are many more neurological conditions which cause similar symptoms, so the clinician should not assume multiple sclerosis is the cause in middle-aged persons presenting with a compatible picture.

多発性硬化症の発症は，ほとんどが若い世代です．このパールは，若いときに発症した患者が，50歳を過ぎてもまだ症状を有しているときの新たな診断についても言及しています．さらに，50歳以降では同じような症状を引き起こすほかの多くの神経疾患があります．ですから，医師は多発性硬化症と一致した臨床像を呈する中年患者の原因を多発性硬化症と決めてかかるべきではありません．

［訳者注］
今回，多発性硬化症が感染症の項目に含まれています．多発性硬化症の原因はいまだ明らかではありませんが，Epstein-Barrウイルス感染が関係している可能性が示唆されています．

NEOPLASTIC DISEASES

腫瘍性疾患

44.

Breast Cancer
乳癌

Denial is extremely common in breast cancer, and should be addressed by all primary care providers.

「乳癌の否認はきわめてありふれている．すべてのプライマリ・ケア従事者が取り組むべき課題である」

Certainly the vast majority of women in the world are well aware of breast cancer, but often choose to ignore the possibility in themselves; any physician in a primary care practice should be aggressive about screening for this appropriately. It remains controversial whether to begin serial screening mammograms at age 40 or age 50, given that breast tissue is quite firm in younger women and thus more likely to produce false-positive results, creating unnecessary anxiety and biopsy procedures.

確かに，世界中のほとんどの女性が乳癌をよく認識しています．しかし，彼女たちは自身の乳癌の可能性を無視しがちです．プライマリ・ケアにおけるすべての医師は，乳癌のスクリーニングを適切な方法で積極的に行うべきです．40〜50歳代の女性への連続的な乳房X線撮影によるスクリーニング開始については，若い女性の硬い乳腺組織が偽陽性を示しがちなため，無用な不安と生検をもたらすので，いまだ議論の余地があります．

45.

Central Nervous System Tumors
中枢神経腫瘍

If a headache awakens a patient from sleep, this condition jumps highly on the list of causes of headache: take this complaint seriously.

「頭痛により患者の眠りが覚めるなら，中枢神経腫瘍が頭痛の原因の上位に跳ね上がる．この訴えは重大ととらえなさい」

Presumably, the increased intravascular volume occurring during recumbency increases intracranial pressure, producing headache which is worse at night. Whether or not this is the reason, this is a symptom that clinicians have long noticed in either primary or metastatic tumors of the brain, of which there are numerous types, most commonly glioblastoma.

おそらく，臥位になったときの血管内の容量増加が頭蓋内圧を上げ，夜間に悪化する頭痛を引き起こすと考えられます．これが機序かどうかはともかく，さまざまなタイプの脳原発腫瘍，もしくは転移性脳腫瘍において，医師は以前からこの症状に気づいていました．なかでも神経膠芽細胞腫は，最も頻度の高いものです．

46.
Cervical Cancer
子宮頸癌

Yet another serious illness preventable by vaccination, this time against human papilloma virus.

「さらにワクチン接種によって防ぎうる他の重大な疾患があった．今回はヒトパピローマウイルスへのワクチン接種である」

It has been determined that the human papilloma virus is the cause of nearly all cases of cervical carcinoma, and if young women are sexually active, vaccination against this virus, although expensive, is well worth the cost. Cervical cancer is also one of a handful of diseases in which strictly defined screening, in this case with Pap smears, has made an important difference in morbidity and mortality.

　ヒトパピローマウイルスは，ほとんどすべての子宮頸癌の原因であることが特定されました．若い女性で性的活動性があるならば，費用はかかるものの，このウイルスに対するワクチン接種には，コストを超える価値があります．子宮頸癌も厳格にスクリーニングが施行されるべき数少ない疾患の1つです．子宮頸癌ではパパニコロウ（Papanicolaou）塗抹試験の施行が，罹患率・死亡率に重要な相違をもたらします．

47.

Colon Cancer
大腸癌

In patients with endocarditis due to Strep bovis, find the tumor; it is most certainly there, given the exceptionally strong association between colonic polyps and carcinoma and this specific form of endocarditis, for reasons remaining somewhat elusive still.

「*Streptococcus bovis* による感染性心内膜炎患者では腫瘍を探しなさい．大腸ポリープや大腸癌とこの特異的な心内膜炎には例外的に強い関係があり，ほとんどの例で腫瘍がみつかる．理由はいまだわかっていない」

A number of years ago it was found that patients with classical subacute bacterial endocarditis had an inordinately high incidence of colonic polyps and adenocarcinoma. Although the has been attributed to translocation of organisms across the damaged colonic wall, other factors must be at play given that no other bacteria are similarly found causing endocarditis in this setting.

　何年も前に，古典的な亜急性心内膜炎の患者が，並外れて高率に大腸ポリープや腺癌を有することがわかりました．*Streptococcus bovis* が傷ついた大腸の粘膜から侵入することが原因と考えられます．しかし，このような状況においては，他の心内膜炎を起こす細菌は認められないため，別の要因があるはずです．

48.
Esophageal Cancer
食道癌

Defined properly, dysphagia is one of the few symptoms in medicine for which an anatomic correlation nearly always is present; too often it is this disease.

「正確に言えば，嚥下困難は，ほぼ常に解剖との関連が存在する数少ない医学上の症状の1つである．食道癌では頻繁に嚥下困難を認める」

The proper definition of dysphagia is difficulty in swallowing, and it does not necessarily imply that pain need be present. The patient typically points to the exact location of the obstruction, and it has been noticed in recent years that adenocarcinoma of the esophagus has become more common, probably due to the oncogenic properties of long-term gastric reflux causing Barrett's esophagus.

嚥下困難の正確な定義は，飲み込むのが難しくなることです．嚥下困難は痛みを伴うことを必ずしも意味しません．患者は，ほぼ正確な閉塞の部位を指し示すことができます．最近，食道の腺癌が増加してきていることがわかってきました．おそらく，長期間の胃食道逆流がバレット食道*を引き起こし，その発癌の特性が原因なのでしょう．

［訳者注］
*バレット食道は重症の逆流性食道炎によって起こる食道扁平上皮から円柱上皮への化生です．

49.

Gastric Carcinoma
胃癌

No acid, no ulcer; 100% of cases of stomach ulcers in achlorhydric patients prove to be malignant.

「酸がなければ,潰瘍はない.無酸症患者の胃潰瘍は100％悪性である」

All peptic disease requires the presence of gastric acid; duodenal ulcers are hypersecretory, and while many gastric ulcers are hyposecretory, it still requires some acid to be present for the formation of a benign ulcer. Stimulation with histamine analogs can determine if the patient has true achlorhydria, since all normal patients increase acid secretion after injection of a low dose of this agent.

すべての消化性潰瘍は,胃酸の存在を必要とします.多くの胃潰瘍では分泌低下を示しますが,十二指腸潰瘍では分泌過剰です.良性の潰瘍の形成には,いくらかの酸の存在が必要なのです.すべての健常者では,少量のヒスタミンアナログ注射後に酸分泌が増加しますので,ヒスタミンアナログによる刺激によって,患者が本当に無酸症であるかを判定できます.

50.

Gestational Trophoblastic Neoplasia
妊娠性栄養膜新生物

Remember this in a woman with severe hyperemesis gravidarum who is also hyperthyroid: beta-hCG has the ability to activate thyroid hormone receptors.

「妊娠性栄養膜新生物はひどい妊娠悪阻と甲状腺機能亢進を伴った患者に認めることを覚えておきなさい．β-hCG は甲状腺ホルモン受容体を活性化する」

This is a most interesting phenomenon, in that the structure of beta-hCG has a small area of amino acid homology with thyroid stimulating hormone. Because patients with gestational tumors, including both hydatidiform mole and choriocarcinoma, have extremely high levels of this gonadotropin, they may stimulate the thyroid hormone receptor enough to cause clinical hyperthyroidism. Rarely, this may be seen even in normal pregnancies.

β-hCG の構造は，わずかな部分に，甲状腺刺激ホルモンのアミノ酸構造と相同性を有しており，これは最も興味深い現象といえるでしょう．胞状奇胎と絨毛癌を含む妊娠腫瘍の患者は，異常に高レベルの性腺刺激ホルモン値を示します．これは甲状腺機能亢進を臨床的に呈するに十分なほど，甲状腺ホルモン受容体を刺激することがあります．この現象は稀に正常妊娠においてさえ認められます．

［訳者注］
妊娠性栄養膜新生物は，胞状奇胎，胎盤部栄養膜腫瘍，絨毛癌を包含する概念です．

51.

Hepatocellular Carcinoma
肝細胞癌

The carrier state for hepatitis B surface antigen, with no liver disease, is a risk factor; in hepatitis C, it is the cirrhosis predisposing to malignant deterioration of the hepatocytes.

「肝疾患のない HBs 抗原キャリアは肝細胞癌の危険因子である．C 型肝炎では肝硬変が肝細胞悪性化の素因になる」

It appears that simply the presence of the hepatitis B virus is oncogenic, and in some patients, this occurs in the absence of historical, physical exam, or laboratory evidence of any liver disease, and indeed, even in those with normal biopsies. In hepatitis C, however, it is similar to other conditions which cause liver cirrhosis, behaving as though the regenerating nodules of cirrhosis may be part of the pathogenesis; however, the carrier state of hepatitis C without clinical disease does not seem to be a risk factor for this extremely common tumor.

B 型肝炎ウイルスの存在は，実際に発癌をもたらします．一部の患者は，病歴，身体所見，検査に肝疾患を示す結果がないにもかかわらず，肝細胞癌を発症します．確かに，肝生検で正常を示す患者においてすら，肝細胞癌の発症をきたすことがあるのです．一方，C 型肝炎では肝硬変を引き起こす他の病態と同様に，まるで肝硬変の再生結節が病因の一部のように推移します．しかし，臨床的に肝炎がない C 型肝炎キャリアの状態は，このきわめて頻度の高い肝細胞癌の危険因子にはならないようです．

52.

Lung Cancer
肺癌

If your patient with COPD develops finger clubbing, obtain a CT scan of the chest; this is the diagnosis.

「慢性閉塞性肺疾患の患者にばち指を認めたら，胸部CTスキャンを撮りなさい．肺癌が診断である」

Digital clubbing, while common in most forms of lung cancer and in other conditions such as congenital heart disease and suppurative lung disease, is not encountered in chronic obstructive pulmonary disease. When it develops, one must have a high index of suspicion for the presence of a lung tumor, which in any event might be expected to occur more commonly in chronic obstructive pulmonary disease because of the relationship of both to cigarette smoking.

ばち指は，ほとんどの型の肺癌，先天性心疾患や化膿性肺疾患で認められます．しかし，慢性閉塞性肺疾患では観察されません．慢性閉塞性疾患と肺癌の両者と喫煙の関係から，慢性閉塞性肺疾患の患者にばち指を認めたら，医師は慢性閉塞性疾患にしばしば合併する肺癌の存在を強く疑わなくてはなりません．

53.

Prostate Cancer
前立腺癌

Screening with PSA is a never-ending argument in this condition; remember that 1% of patients have a small cell carcinoma of the prostate, and therefore have normal PSA levels.

「PSA による前立腺癌スクリーニングは終わりなき論争である．前立腺癌の 1% の患者は小細胞癌であり，それゆえ PSA は正常であることを覚えておきなさい」

As the population of older men increases throughout the world, a coherent strategy for screening for this tumor is essential. It appears that certain groups, such as younger African American men, have a much more aggressive course; however, once past age 70, it is highly debatable whether treatment prolongs life, and certainly prostatectomy at any age is associated with numerous unappealing side effects due to denervation of the genitourinary system.

世界中で高齢男性の人口が増加していますので，前立腺癌スクリーニングの一貫した戦略は必須です．アフリカ系米国人の若年男性といった一部のグループの前立腺癌は，かなり侵襲的な経過をたどります．しかし，いったん 70 歳を過ぎると，治療が生存期間を延長するのかどうか，論争の余地がでてきます．どのような年齢層における前立腺摘除術も，泌尿生殖器系の除神経による歓迎されない多くの後遺症を確かにもたらしますから．

54.

Renal Cell Carcinoma
腎細胞癌

The internist's tumor: numerous perineoplastic phenomena occur in this disease, often mimicking conditions far from the kidney.

「腎細胞癌は内科医の腫瘍である．数多くの傍腫瘍現象がこの疾患で起こる．腎臓由来とは思えない症状が多い」

For reasons both known and unknown, renal cell carcinoma's remote effects are numerous; perhaps most notable is the hepatopathy with its elevated alkaline phosphatase that disappears upon removal of the tumor. Other features include erythrocytosis, recurrence after decades of apparent clinical cure, hypercalcemia, and even hypoglycemia.

機序は明らかであったり，不明であったりですが，腎細胞癌の遠隔臓器への影響は数多くあります．おそらく，最も気づかれるのが，アルカリフォスファターゼ値上昇を伴う肝障害でしょう．これは腫瘍の摘出により改善します．他には，赤血球増加，明らかな臨床的治癒後，数十年しての再発，高カルシウム血症，低血糖すら起こりえます．

55.
Testicular Cancer
精巣癌

The number one cause of a malignancy in a man between 20 and 35; ordinarily, the patient notices the responsible lesion himself, and comes to the physician thereafter.

「20〜35歳の男性患者の悪性腫瘍の最も多い原因は精巣腫瘍である．通常，患者自身が責任病変に気づき，その後医師のもとを訪れる」

Although it may appear somewhat draconian, unilateral orchiectomy is necessary to diagnose this tumor, given the risk of tracking tumor cells back along a biopsy needle's route; the patient maintains fertility, however, and in the modern day, virtually all are curable, even tumors metastatic at presentation.

生検には腫瘍細胞が生検針の侵入路に沿って播種するリスクがあるため，いくぶん苛酷と眼に映るかもしれませんが，精巣腫瘍を診断するためには片側の睾丸摘除術が必要です．患者は生殖力を維持できます．今日では，実質的にすべての例で，診断時に腫瘍が転移していたとしても治癒が見込めます．

HEMATOLOGIC TUMORS

血液悪性腫瘍

56.

Acute Leukemia
急性白血病

Pain radiating down the legs can simulate disk herniation in this disease, but is in fact caused expanding bone marrow.

「急性白血病では下肢に放散する痛みが椎間板ヘルニアに酷似するかもしれない．しかし，事実は骨髄の膨張による」

This disorder has a fairly short symptomatic period before patients seek care, and one of the characteristic symptoms is related to the replacement of bone marrow by rapidly multiplying tumor cells; when this occurs in the femoral marrow, the clinician may be fooled into thinking that there may be mechanical low back disease, such as spinal stenosis or bilateral disk herniation.

急性白血病では患者が医療機関を受診する前に，症状を有するほんの短い期間があります．1つの特徴的な症状は，急速に増殖する腫瘍細胞によって骨髄が置き換わってしまうことに関連しています．これが大腿骨の骨髄で起こると，医師は脊柱管狭窄症，両側の椎間板ヘルニアのようなメカニカルな腰の疾患を鑑別診断として考えてしまい，だまされることがあります．

57.

Chronic Lymphocytic Leukemia
慢性リンパ性白血病

Smudge cells are noted on the peripheral blood smear in this condition; this is an artifact of the staining process, not an intrinsic abnormality of the cell.

「染みのついた細胞が慢性リンパ性白血病の末梢血スメアで観察される．これは細胞の内因性の異常ではなく染色過程の人工的産物である」

Upon occasion, clinicians may see large numbers of what appear to be possibly mitotic nuclei in an otherwise stable patient with chronic lymphatic leukemia. In fact, they are smudge cells, which occur during the smearing and staining of the blood, and are of little clinical significance.

ときおり，医師は安定した慢性リンパ性白血病の患者において，有糸分裂中の核と思われる染みのついた数多くの細胞をみつけるかもしれません．実際，染みがついた細胞であり，これはスメアをひき，血液を染色している間に起こります．臨床的重要性はほとんどありません．

58.

Chronic Myelogenous Leukemia
慢性骨髄性白血病

If a patient with this disorder has a blood glucose of zero without symptoms, it is an artifact.

「慢性骨髄性白血病の患者が症状のない血糖値0を呈したら，それは人工的産物である」

Pseudohypoglycemia occurs in patients with exceptionally high neutrophil counts, which are typical of this condition; what occurs is *in vitro* metabolism after phlebotomy, the blood cells consuming the glucose in the plasma while awaiting processing by the lab. Thus, when the plasma is finally tested for glucose concentration, it will be zero, despite the absence of symptoms of hypoglycemia.

偽性低血糖は慢性骨髄性白血病において，典型的に好中球が並外れて増加している患者に起こります．採血後から測定を待っている間に，血球が血漿の糖を消費してしまう試験管内での代謝に原因があります．このように，患者には症状が全くないにもかかわらず，最終的に血漿の糖濃度が測定される段階で，血糖値0という結果が示されます．

59.

Essential Thrombocytosis
本態性血小板増加症

Clotting and bleeding disorders in this condition are not related to the platelet count, but to qualitative abnormalities in these cells.

「本態性血小板増加症において凝固し出血する病態は,血小板数でなく,血小板の質的異常に関連する」

　Platelets are sufficiently small that even in situations where normal platelets are markedly elevated, the rheology of the blood is not affected, and thus, no abnormal clotting occurs. In essential thrombocytosis, there are functional, as well as numerical, abnormalities of the platelets, so patients with this condition both bleed and clot abnormally.

　正常な血小板であれば,どんなに数が増えたとしても,その大きさは十分に小さく,血液の流体力学には影響を及ぼしません.ですから,異常な凝固は起こりません.本態性血小板増加症には,血小板数と同様に血小板の機能的な異常があります.このため本態性血小板増加症の患者では,出血と凝固の異常が起こるのです.

60.

Hodgkin's Disease
ホジキン病

If a patient develops chest pain shortly after drinking alcohol, this may be the diagnosis; be sure to obtain chest imaging on such patients.

「アルコール摂取後間もなく胸痛を訴える患者では，ホジキン病の可能性がある．胸部画像検査を行いなさい」

Although Hodgkin's disease is now appreciably less common than non-Hodgkin's lymphoma, it is still potentially curable. A rare but characteristic symptom very typical of this condition is pain in affected lymph nodes after drinking alcohol. The causes of this are unknown, but when present, the clinician must have a high index of suspicion for this disease.

今日，ホジキン病は非ホジキンリンパ腫に比べかなり稀な疾患ですが，きちんと治療すれば治癒可能です．ホジキン病において，稀ながらも，きわめて典型的で特徴的な症状は，アルコール摂取後に影響を受けているリンパ節に起こる痛みなのです．機序は不明ですが，もしも，この症状を認めたときは，医師はホジキン病を強く疑わなければなりません．

61.

Multiple Myeloma
多発性骨髄腫

The three unexpected no's of myeloma: no fever, no increased alkaline phosphatase, and no splenomegaly.

「多発性骨髄腫では期待しない3つのノー（なし）がある．発熱なし，アルカリフォスファターゼの上昇なし，脾腫なし」

Most hematologic tumors are characterized by fever, but its presence in myeloma indicates an associated infection. Similarly, splenomegaly, typical of other hematologic malignancies, is not present in myeloma. Finally, despite extensive involvement of the skeleton, the alkaline phosphatase level is normal, this being due to the fact that myeloma lesions are purely osteolytic.

ほとんどの血液悪性腫瘍は，発熱により特徴づけられます．しかし，多発性骨髄腫に発熱を認めた場合，それは感染症の合併を示唆します．同様に，他の血液悪性腫瘍に典型的な脾腫も，多発性骨髄腫には存在しません．最後に，広範な骨病変にもかかわらず，アルカリフォスファターゼ値は正常を示します．これは骨髄腫の骨病変が純粋に骨溶性であること*に由来します．

［訳者注］
*骨溶性でも骨形成が促進する病態（例：癌の骨転移）では，アルカリフォスファターゼ値が上昇します．

62.

Non-Hodgkin's Lymphoma
非ホジキンリンパ腫

Despite the clinical stage, the assumption is made in all patients with non-Hodgkin's lymphoma that the disease is systemic at the time of diagnosis, and treated as such.

「病期に関係なく，非ホジキンリンパ腫と診断されたすべての患者において，疾患は診断時に全身的でそれに沿った治療が必要と推測される」

The majority of patients with Hodgkin's lymphoma behave as though the tumor starts in one lymph node, and spreads in an orderly fashion to contiguous groups. In the increasingly more common non-Hodgkin's lymphoma, however, the clinical behavior suggests a multifocal origin, and as such, the majority of patients with it are treated systemically with chemotherapy; flow cytometry has helped elucidate the pathogenesis and correct treatment of this condition.

ほとんどのホジキンリンパ腫患者では，あたかも腫瘍は1つのリンパ節から始まり，整然と隣接するリンパ節群に広がるようにみえます．しかし，増加している非ホジキンリンパ腫患者の臨床経過を観察すると，多病巣性の起源が示唆され，大半の非ホジキンリンパ腫の患者には，化学療法による全身的な治療が行われます．フローサイトメトリーは，病因の明瞭化，正しい治療法の選択に役立ちます．

63.

Paroxysmal Nocturnal Hemoglobinuria
発作性夜間ヘモグロビン尿症

No other condition in medicine has hypercoagulability associated with pancytopenia.

「発作性夜間ヘモグロビン尿症以外に汎血球減少を合併し過凝固を呈する医学上の疾患はない」

PNH is an interesting and pleomorphic condition, and in many patients, pancytopenia is encountered. For reasons that are not clear scientifically, rather than being associated with abnormal bleeding, in fact hypercoagulability is the rule, particularly in intraabdominal veins.

発作性夜間ヘモグロビン尿症は興味深い多型性な疾患で,多くの患者が汎血球減少を呈します.その興味深さは異常な出血を合併することよりも,科学的に明らかになっておらず,事実,過凝固が常に存在し,それが腹腔内の静脈に特異的だからです.

64. Polycythemia Vera
真性赤血球症

The only disease in medicine with iron deficiency despite polycythemia.

「多血にもかかわらず鉄欠乏を認める医学上の唯一の疾患は真性赤血球症である」

In this myeloproliferative condition, the dominantly affected cell is the erythrocyte, and it expands clonally until the body runs out of iron; thus, one may observe a remarkably elevated hemoglobin and hematocrit, yet have clinical studies associated with iron deficiency. Like the other myeloproliferative conditions, polycythemia vera also has an elevated serum B_{12} level, splenomegaly, and an abnormal mutation, in this case, it being JAK2.

この骨髄増殖性疾患において，主に影響を受けるのは赤血球です．生体の鉄を消費し尽くすまで，赤血球がクローン性に増殖します．このように，医師は著明に増加したヘモグロビンとヘマトクリットにもかかわらず，鉄欠乏を合併していることを観察するでしょう．他の骨髄増殖性疾患と同様に，真性赤血球症では，ビタミン B_{12} の上昇，脾腫，異常な V617F 変異である JAK2 陽性を認めます．

65.

Waldenström's Macroglobulinemia
マクログロブリン血症

There's rouleaux and then there's rouleaux; some is found on every blood smear, but in this disorder, nearly every erythrocyte appears to be one of a stack of dishes.

「連銭形成,そして連銭形成.どんな血液像でもいくつか見つかる.しかし,マクログロブリン血症ではほとんどすべての赤血球が皿を積み重ねたように見える」

It is usual to observe occasional groups of erythrocytes appear to be in small stacks when reviewing a normal peripheral blood smear; however, the paraprotein in this condition, as well as in multiple myeloma, in many cases results in the majority of red cells appearing in this conformity. Thus, to be significant, rouleaux formation must be encountered on virtually every field of inspection of the peripheral blood.

正常の末梢血液像を見ていると,一部の赤血球が小さく積み重なった様に認められることが稀ではありません.しかし,マクログロブリン血症の異常蛋白は,多発性骨髄腫と同様に多くの例で,ほとんどすべての赤血球に連銭形成をもたらします.このように,特異的に,末梢血液像のほとんどの視野に連銭形成が必ず認められます.

RHEUMATOLOGY
自己免疫性疾患

66.

Adult Still's Disease
成人スティル病

In a patient with fever of unknown origin which has escaped diagnosis, look carefully for the pink truncal rash during fever spikes; this is the diagnosis.

「診断がつかない不明熱の患者では,スパイク状の発熱時にピンクの体幹の発疹がでないか注意深く観察しなさい.あれば成人スティル病が診断である」

This disease is being increasingly recognized, and remains a diagnosis of exclusion; there is no significant test consistently positive, except perhaps the serum ferritin, itself non-specific. Given all the negative cultures, biopsies, and serological markers, it may be said to be the great masquerader of the 21st century.

成人スティル病はよく認識されるようになってきました.また,いまだに除外診断が必要です.おそらく,フェリチン以外に一貫して陽性を示す特異的検査はなく,フェリチンそのものも非特異的です.血液培養,生検,血清学的マーカー,すべて陰性で,21世紀における主要なる「仮面舞踏会の参加者」といえます.

［訳者注］
「仮面舞踏会の参加者」(masquerader) はいくつもの鑑別診断が挙がる,診断の難しい疾患の比喩としてよく用いられます.虫垂炎も1つの masquerader といえる疾患でしょう.

67.

Ankylosing Spondylitis
強直性脊椎炎

Two underappreciated late complications: an idiopathic apical pulmonary fibrosis simulating TB, and a cauda equina syndrome resembling structural disease in the lower spinal cord.

「強直性脊椎炎には2つのあまり知られていない晩期の合併症がある．1つは結核に似る特発性肺尖部線維症であり，もう1つは下部脊髄の構造的な疾患に似る馬尾症候群である」

This condition, seen more often in patients with the HLA-B27 histocompatibility antigen, in its early phases presents as a backache and peripheral arthritis in young men. For reasons thoroughly unknown, many years after the arthritis has burned out, sterile biapical pulmonary cavities can be encountered, as may be fibrosis of the cauda equina. Thus, if a patient with either of these conditions has a past history of unexplained back pain and arthritis, do not (1) treat for tuberculosis which is not present, or (2) perform surgery on the prostate because of urinary retention.

強直性脊椎炎はHLA-B27陽性の若い男性患者によく認められます．初期には背部痛，末梢の関節炎が認められます．機序は完全にはわかっていませんが，何年も経て関節炎が燃え尽きた後，無菌性の両側肺尖部の囊胞性病変，また，馬尾の線維化を認めることがあります．ですから，両肺尖部の囊胞性病変と馬尾症候群の患者で過去に説明のつかない背部痛，関節炎の既往がある場合は，（1）結核でないのに結核の治療を，（2）尿閉のために前立腺の手術をしないでください．

68.

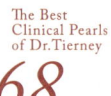

Arthritis Associated with Inflammatory Bowel Disease
炎症性腸疾患に伴う関節炎

Arthritis in adolescence commonly has the physician suspicious for sexually transmitted diseases; be careful not to miss IBD as the cause, as younger patients have a tendency not to complain about bowel symptoms.

「青年期の関節炎では一般に医師は性行為感染症（STD）による関節炎*を疑う．しかし，炎症性腸疾患が原因である関節炎を見落とさないこと．若い炎症性腸疾患の患者では腸の症状を訴えない傾向がある」

The association of both types of IBD with arthritis has long been known. If patients who are HLA-B27-positive contract IBD, nearly all will develop ankylosing spondylitis. More common is an inflammatory, symmetrical polyarthritis very similar to rheumatoid disease, but notable for its lack of seropositivity.

　潰瘍性大腸炎，クローン（Crohn）病の2つの炎症性腸疾患と関節炎の関係は以前から知られていました．HLA-B27陽性の患者が炎症性腸疾患に罹患したら，ほとんどすべての患者が強直性脊椎炎を発症します．炎症の強い，対称性の多関節炎を呈することが多く，関節リウマチに酷似しますが，血清反応陰性であることに注目します．

［訳者注］
*クラミジアによる関節炎，無菌性尿道炎，結膜炎のことです．

69.

Behçet's Disease
ベーチェット病

A stroke in a young Japanese woman is Behçet's until proven otherwise.

「若い日本人女性の脳卒中では他の診断がつくまでベーチェット病を考えなさい」

This disorder is found along the famous "Silk Route" from Turkey to the Far East, and while painful oral and genital ulcers are the most common manifestations, a vasculitis causing a stroke, particularly in young women, is its most feared association. Interestingly, markers of inflammation are seldom markedly abnormal in this difficult-to-treat condition.

ベーチェット病はトルコから極東までの有名な「シルクロード」に沿って認められます．有痛性の口腔内・陰部潰瘍が最も頻度の高い症状ですが，血管炎は特に若い女性に最もおそろしい合併症である脳卒中を引き起こします．興味深いことに，この治療が困難な病態では，炎症のマーカーが稀にしか異常値を示しません．

70.

Carpal Tunnel Syndrome
手根管症候群

Though the lesion is at the wrist, the pain may go all the way back up the arm in the median nerve distribution... and the clinician hopes it's on the right side.

「手根管症候群の病変は手首にあるが，疼痛は正中神経の分布に沿って腕まで上行することがある．臨床医は右手にそれが起こることを願う」

Carpal tunnel syndrome may mimic a cervical radiculopathy, and of more concern, myocardial ischemia or infarction. Two points of interest: (1) the pain of carpal tunnel is consistently worse at night, and (2) the discomfort involves the thumb, index, and long fingers, whereas myocardial pain affects the ring and small fingers.

手根管症候群は頸椎の神経根障害に似ることがあります．さらに，心筋虚血，もしくは心筋梗塞にも似ることがあるのです．興味深いのは2つの点です．（1）手根管症候群の疼痛は，一貫して夜間に悪化します．（2）不快感は拇指・示指・中指に認めます．一方，心筋由来の疼痛は，（左の）環指・小指に起こります．

71. Pseudogout
偽痛風

Chondrocalcinosis is the radiological finding; pseudogout is the clinical association.

「軟骨石灰化症はX線上の所見である．偽痛風は臨床的な症状である」

While many patients with attacks of pseudogout—a crystalline arthritis with strongly positive birefringent crystals under polarizing microscopy—it is not necessary to have calcification of the cartilage to make this diagnosis. It is a more indolent disorder than gout, and it is to be remembered that chondrocalcinosis may be seen in degenerative arthritis with few or no symptoms.

偽痛風の発作の患者の多くは，偏光顕微鏡下で複屈折する結晶が強陽性の結晶誘発性関節炎ですが，診断には必ずしも軟骨の石灰化を必要とはしません．偽痛風は痛風に比べ，痛みは軽いことが多いのです．軟骨石灰化症は，症状が少ないか，全くない変性による関節炎に認められることを覚えておいてください．

［訳者注］
　膝の変形性関節症においても，軟骨の石灰化をときに認めます．

72.

Vasculitis
血管炎

It is vasculitis until proven otherwise if your patient has: palpable purpura; unexplained neuropathy; glomerulonephritis; ischemic symptomatology at a young age; FUO, or unexplained polysystem disease.

「あなたの患者が,触れる紫斑,説明のつかない神経炎,糸球体腎炎,若年における虚血症状,不明熱,もしくは説明のつかない多臓器病変を呈していたら他の診断がつくまで血管炎を考えなさい」

Many beginning clinicians find vasculitis to be confusing, and difficult to classify. In fact, the role of the primary provider is merely to identify whether vasculitis is present, and the above pearl lists many, if not all, of the characteristic findings. Once identified, then more specialized providers can advise as regards classification, treatment and, if known, cause.

多くの若い医師は,血管炎の診断は紛らわしく,分類が困難と思われるでしょう.事実,プライマリ・ケア医の役割は,単に血管炎の存在を見極めることにあります.上記のパールは,すべてではありませんが,血管炎の多くの特徴的な症状について記述しています.いったん,血管炎と診断できたら,専門医が血管炎の分類,治療,わかれば原因についての助言をしてくれるでしょう.

73.

Cryoglobulinemia
クリオグロブリン血症

When the laboratory tells you the CBC has "clotted" it may not be a clot, but a gel effect in the plasma caused by a monoclonal spike.

「検査室から血算が凝固してしまったと報告があったときは，それは凝固でなく，単クローン性免疫グロブリン増加による血漿のゲル効果である」

　Cryoglobulinemia comes in several forms, perhaps most notably as a cryoprecipitable immune complex as part of the hepatitis C vasculitis complex. However, any elevated globulin, particularly the monoclonal proteins of myeloma and macroglobulinemia, has this property. Remember that although the prefix "cryo" refers to cold, the temperature of the body is 37 degrees Celsius, and thus, even room temperature is relatively "cold" in comparison to body temperature, and thus precipitates the protein.

　クリオグロブリン血症にはいくつかの型があります．とりわけ多いのは，C型肝炎による本態性混合型クリオグロブリン血症の寒冷で沈降をきたす免疫複合体です．しかし，特に骨髄腫とマクログロブリン血症における単クローン性の免疫グロブリン，および上昇しているどんな免疫グロブリンでも，この血漿のゲル効果を有しています．クリオグロブリン血症の最初の「クリオ」という言葉は，寒冷に関連した意味ですが，体温は37℃ということを覚えておいてください．室内温ですら体温に比べれば相対的に「寒冷」なのです．このように蛋白が沈殿します．

［訳者注］
　クリオグロブリン血症は，紫斑・多関節痛・ニューロパチー・糸球体腎炎を特徴とする血管炎を伴うことがあります．Ⅰ型は単クローン性で骨髄腫とマクログロブリン血症によります．混合型クリオグロブリン血症には，多クローン性IgGと単クローン性IgMからなるⅡ型，多クローン性IgGとIgMからなるⅢ型があります．C型肝炎はⅡ型を呈します．

74.

Fibromyalgia
線維筋痛症

If your patient complains of tenderness each time you touch them during an exam, this is probably the diagnosis; however, be certain the CRP and ESR are normal before saying so.

「診察中,触れるたびに圧痛を訴える患者では,診断はおそらく線維筋痛症である.しかし,診断する前に,CRP・血沈正常が前提である」

There has been a lot of interest in the media about this condition, which appears to debilitate the young women whom it affects preferentially, yet all objective signs of inflammation are absent. This, in turn, has led some to believe that other factors besides immunological abnormalities may be responsible. It is safe to say, however, that this disorder is not life-threatening and does not produce anatomic disability.

線維筋痛症については多くの関心がメディアのなかにあります.線維筋痛症は特に若い女性に多く,彼女たちを衰弱させます.にもかかわらず,炎症の客観的徴候がありません.次に考えられることは,免疫学的な異常以外のほかの因子が原因かもしれないということです.しかし,線維筋痛症は生命を脅かす疾患ではなく,解剖学的な障害も起こさないといって差し支えないでしょう.

75.

Gout
痛風

With repeated attacks, this condition becomes increasingly symmetrical and polyarticular; however, if it involves the hips or shoulders, make a different diagnosis.

「痛風発作をくり返すと，関節炎は対称性の多関節炎となる．しかし，股関節炎，もしくは肩関節炎を認めたら，ほかの疾患である」

Initial attacks of gout are classical monoarticular, nocturnal, and associated with a red and extremely tender joint. With time, however, with the accumulation of tophi in many parts of the body and with arthritis in increasing numbers of joints, it may resemble other destructive types of arthritis. The relatively warmer temperature of the deeper hips and shoulders make precipitation of uric acid crystals much less likely. This process favors more distal joints such as the first metatarsal-phalangeal.

　初回の痛風発作は，夜間に起こり，発赤し，強い圧痛を伴う古典的な単関節炎です．しかし，時間を経ると，体のあちこちに痛風結節が形成され，関節炎を起こす部位が増え，関節破壊を起こすほかの関節炎に似てきます．体の深部にある肩・股関節は，ほかの関節に比べ比較的温度が高く，尿酸の析出が起こりくいのです．尿酸の析出は，比較的温度の低い第 1 中足趾節間関節のような，より遠位の関節に起こりやすいのです．

76.

Hypersensitivity Vasculitis
過敏性血管炎

The telltale lesion of this condition is dependent purpura; thus, while typically on the legs, be sure to examine the back in patients who are chronically bedbound.

「過敏性血管炎の証拠となる病変は紫斑である．足に起こるのが典型であるが，長期臥床している患者では背中の診察を必ず行いなさい」

This is a small-vessel vasculitis, most often due to a drug reaction or to association with hepatitis C and cryoglobulinemia, but remains confined to the skin, rarely causing concerns such as nervous system or large-vessel involvement.

過敏性血管炎は小血管炎で，薬剤の副作用，C型肝炎，クリオグロブリン血症が原因のことが多いのです．しかし，これは皮膚に限局し，神経，もしくは大血管に障害は起こしません．

［訳者注］
過敏性血管炎は皮膚血管炎（cutaneous vasculitis）とも呼ばれます．

77.

Microscopic Polyangiitis
顕微鏡的多発動脈炎

As in so many suspected cases of vasculitis, tissue is the issue as regards establishing a diagnosis.

「血管炎を疑う多くの患者が存在する．診断の確立には組織が問題である」

While there are many different types of vasculitis, both pathologically and clinically, as well as differences in the pattern of positive autoantibodies encountered, to be certain of the approach to proper treatment one should establish a tissue diagnosis.

　病理学的，臨床的に異なるいくつものタイプの血管炎があり，同様に自己抗体陽性のパターンの違いにも遭遇します．適切な治療を選択するためには，組織での診断を確立する必要があります．

[訳者注]
　日本では高齢者の顕微鏡的多発動脈炎が稀ではありません．抗好中球細胞質ミエロペルオキシダーゼ抗体（myeloperoxidase antineutrophic cytoplasmic antibodies: MPO-ANCA）の測定，多発性単神経炎を呈する患者では神経生検，蛋白尿，血尿，腎機能障害を呈する患者では腎生検を行います．小血管にフィブリノイド壊死，もしくは半月体形成性糸球体腎炎の所見を認めます．
　Tissue is the issue は組織所見が診断にとって欠かせないときのパールです．

78.

Osteomyelitis
骨髄炎

Once an osteo, always an osteo.

「一度骨髄炎に罹患したら，常に骨髄炎の可能性がある」

　This applies to osteomyelitis in bones, such as those in the foot, where circulation can be poor with peripheral vascular disease Likewise, in diabetics as well, osteomyelitis is an indolent condition which may be extremely difficult both to diagnose and to eradicate. The acute osteomyelitis of younger persons should in fact not be so difficult to cure.

　このパールは，末梢の血管病変により，循環の低下した足の骨髄炎に適応できます．同様に，糖尿病では，診断と根治がきわめて難しい無痛性の骨髄炎を呈します．逆に，若年者の急性骨髄炎は，事実，治癒が困難ではありません．

79.

Polyarteritis Nodosa
結節性多発動脈炎

If a patient with cholecystitis shows hints of systemic illness, it may well be cystic artery vasculitis causing the problem.

「胆嚢炎患者が全身的な疾患の可能性を示したら，結節性多発動脈炎による胆嚢動脈炎が胆嚢炎を起こしているかもしれない」

A polyarteritis in its usual iteration is a disorder of medium-sized vessels, and in upwards of 80% of individuals, affects arteries in the intestinal circulation; for reasons not entirely understood, the cystic artery in particular is favored by this pathologic process, resulting in otherwise typical cholecystitis in the absence of gallbladder calculi, referred to as acalculous cholecystitis.

結節性多発動脈炎はくり返す多発動脈炎で中型血管の異常です．80％以上の患者の腸循環にかかわる血管に影響が及びます．機序は完全にわかっていませんが，特異的に胆嚢動脈にこの病的な過程が起こりやすく，結果的に典型的な胆石のない胆嚢炎が起こり，無石胆嚢炎としてとらえられます．

［訳者注］
アメリカリウマチ学会による結節性多発動脈炎の診断基準
① 4 kg 以上の体重減少，② 網状皮斑，③ 睾丸痛，または圧痛，④ 筋痛，筋力低下，下肢の圧痛，⑤ 単神経炎，または多発性単神経炎，⑥ 拡張期血圧 90 mmHg 以上，⑦ BUN 40 mg/dL 以上，または Cr 1.5 mg/dL 以上，⑧ B 型肝炎の抗原，または抗体陽性，⑨ 動脈造影での動脈瘤，閉塞所見，⑩ 生検組織での中小動脈の血管炎
以上の 10 項目のうち 3 項目以上満たすものを結節性多発動脈炎と診断する（感度 82％，特異度 87％）．

80.

Polymyalgia Rheumatica
リウマチ性多発筋痛症

Likely the only condition in medicine for which the erythrocyte sedimentation rate enjoys diagnostic value.

「血沈が診断的価値に恵まれる医学上の唯一の疾患は，リウマチ性多発筋痛症である」

Polymyalgia Rheumatica, which is well-named because of the symptoms of proximal muscle pain and stiffness, is similar in certain respects to fibromyalgia. However, it is not uncommon for patients with PMR to have sedimentation rates in excess of 100, and in 20%, there is an association with giant cell arteritis. There is NO muscle weakness or elevation of CK.

近位筋の痛み・こわばりは，線維筋痛症にかなり似るため，リウマチ性多発筋痛症という病名は症状をよく表現しています．しかし，リウマチ性多発筋痛症では，血沈が 100 mm/時間を超えることが稀ではなく，20%の患者では，巨細胞性動脈炎を合併します．筋力低下，クレアチンキナーゼの上昇がないことが重要なポイントです．

[訳者注]
　リウマチ性多発筋痛症の患者に筋力低下はありませんが，徒手筋力テストの際には，疼痛・こわばりのために，特に三角筋，上腕の筋群に力が入らず正確な評価ができないことを覚えておいてください．
　一方，血沈の正常値(mm/時間)は
男性：年齢÷2
女性：(年齢＋10)÷2
と覚えます．

81.

Psoriatic Arthritis
乾癬性関節炎

In some cases, the psoriasis may be hidden in the intergluteal folds or the umbilicus; be sure to exam the skin thoroughly in an unexplained seronegative arthritis.

「乾癬の病変はときに臀裂，もしくは臍部に隠れることがある．説明のつかない血清反応陰性の関節炎では皮膚をくまなく診察しなさい」

Psoriasis may be associated with a number of different types of arthritis, the most classical involving the distal interphalangeal joints only; a peripheral seronegative arthritis and, in some, sacroiliitis may be present. While the course of the arthritis may parallel that of the cutaneous abnormalities, in certain instances, the psoriatic lesions may be difficult to find, and are present in parts of the skin which are ordinarily not examined, especially in overweight patients.

　乾癬はいくつかの異なるタイプの関節炎を合併します．古典的な遠位指節間関節に限局する関節炎が最も多く，さらに血清反応陰性の末梢の関節炎をきたすものがあり，仙腸関節炎をきたすものもあります．関節炎の経過は，皮膚の症状と並行して推移することがありますが，ときに乾癬の病変はみつけるのが難しく，通常は診察しない場所に病変が存在することがあります．特に肥満患者では注意して診察してください．

82.

Rheumatoid Arthritis
関節リウマチ

In a patient with established rheumatoid arthritis, a flare-up of a single joint while others are stable is a septic arthritis until proven otherwise.

「関節リウマチの診断が確立した患者において、ほかの関節症状が安定しているにもかかわらず、単関節のみが再燃したら、ほかの診断がつくまで感染性関節炎を考えなさい」

The pace of rheumatoid arthritis tends to be that of a symmetrical arthropathy in which all involved joints flare and remit over time. If an otherwise well-treated patient with this disorder exacerbates a single joint, the clinician must be alert to the possibility of infection, insofar as it is a common complication of rheumatoid arthritis requiring immediate attention.

関節リウマチの経過は、影響を受けている関節が再燃と寛解を経時的にくり返す対称性関節炎です。比較的よく治療されている関節リウマチ患者において単関節のみ悪化したときは、医師は感染の可能性に注意しなければいけません。感染性関節炎は迅速な対応が必要な、関節リウマチに頻度の多い合併症です。

83.

Sjögren's Syndrome
シェーグレン症候群

Although a legitimate medical problem, you will see one Sjögren's syndrome in every 50 patients who complain of dry mouth.

「口腔内乾燥は正当な医学的症候であるが，口腔内乾燥を訴える 50 人の患者のうちの 1 人がシェーグレン症候群である」

　Xerostomia is an extremely common primary care complaint, and the appreciable majority of patients with it do not have Sjögren's syndrome. Often, pilocarpine is given to improve salivary secretions, but on occasion, this drug causes enlargement of those glands, mimicking an enlarged lymph node or even a parotid tumor.

　口腔内乾燥症はプライマリ・ケアにおいて，とても頻度の多い訴えです．そして，口腔内乾燥症患者のほとんどは，シェーグレン症候群ではありません．ピロカルピン（ムスカリン受容体刺激薬）が唾液分泌改善のためによく用いられます．ときに，この薬剤は唾液腺を腫脹させ，リンパ節腫脹，もしくは耳下腺腫瘍にすら似た所見を呈します．

84.

Systemic Lupus Erythematosus
全身性エリテマトーデス

A scourge of young women, particularly common in Asia, with a worse prognosis when kidney or central nervous system are involved.

「全身性エリテマトーデスは若い女性の災難である．特にアジアに多い．腎臓と中枢神経ループスの予後は悪い」

Criteria for the diagnosis of SLE are well-established, but on occasion, less than 4 of the 11 criteria are not present at the time of initial diagnosis; similarly, low titer of antinuclear antibody (ANA) is present in a number of patients without this very protean disorder.

全身性エリテマトーデスの診断基準*はよく確立されたものですが，ときに，最初の診断時には，11項目のうち4つ未満の項目しか満たさないことがあります．同様に，さまざまな症状を呈するこの疾患ではないのに，抗核抗体が低いタイターを示す患者は少なくありません．

［訳者注］
*この診断基準は特異度が高く感度は低いのです．
全身性エリテマトーデスの診断基準
①頬部紅斑，②円板状紅斑，③光線過敏症，④口腔内潰瘍，⑤関節炎，⑥漿膜炎，⑦腎障害，⑧神経障害，⑨血液学的所見（溶血性貧血，白血球減少，血小板減少），⑩免疫学的所見（抗DNA抗体，抗Sm抗体，抗リン脂質抗体），⑪抗核抗体
観察期間中，経時的あるいは同時に，11項目のうち4項目以上が存在するとき，全身性エリテマトーデスと診断する（感度75％，特異度95％）．
　低感度，高特異度ということは，その疾患であるのに否定される（偽陰性）可能性が潜んでいます．

85.

Systemic Sclerosis (Scleroderma)
全身性強皮症(強皮症)

Remember CREST: Calcinosis, Raynaud's, Esophageal abnormalities, Sclerodactyly, and periungual Telangiectasias.

「石灰化,レイノー現象,食道の異常,強指症,爪周囲の毛細血管拡張の頭文字,CREST症候群を覚えておきなさい」

While a majority of patients has a limited form of this disease, about one patient in five will have serious interstitial lung disease or renal involvement with difficult-to-control hypertension; mortality rates in patients with more systemic disease tend to be higher during cold winters.

多くの患者は限局型全身性強皮症です.強皮症患者5人に1人は,重篤な間質性肺疾患,もしくはコントロール困難な高血圧をきたす腎クリーゼを有します.さらに,全身的病変を有する患者では,寒い冬に死亡率が上昇します.

[訳者注]
　全身性強皮症は大きく2つに分類されます.皮膚硬化が手から前腕にとどまる限局型全身性強皮症と,その他の部位にも皮膚硬化が及ぶ,びまん型全身性強皮症です.CREST症候群は限局型全身性強皮症で典型的に認められます.全身性強皮症では肺高血圧症の合併にも注意が必要です.

86.

Takayasu's Arteritis
高安動脈炎

Difficult to diagnose early, easy to diagnose late.

「高安動脈炎の早期診断は困難であり，晩期の診断はやさしい」

Takayasu's, sometimes called Pulseless Disease, evolves in a more or less consistent fashion, starting with nonspecific systemic symptoms with elevated markers of inflammation, slowly progressing through increasing arterial insufficiency, with, ultimately, noninflammatory fibrosis of involved arteries, usually of the upper extremities. Thus, blood pressure in the arms may be low enough to cause the radial pulses to be absent.

高安動脈炎はときに脈なし病と呼ばれます．多かれ少なかれ，一貫した経過で病状は進行します．炎症性マーカーの上昇を伴う非特異的な全身症状から始まり，動脈の灌流不全がゆっくりと進行します．最終的には炎症所見の消失した動脈の線維化をきたします．これは上肢に起こりやすいのです．このように，橈骨動脈の拍動が触れなくなるに十分なほど，上腕の血圧が低下します．

［訳者注］
　金沢医学専門学校（現金沢大学医学部）眼科教授の高安右人（1860～1936年）が明治41年（1908年）に，眼底に花環状の血管吻合と血管瘤様の変化を認めた21歳女性を「奇異なる網膜血管の変状に就いて」として報告しました．これが「高安病」と呼ばれる疾患概念確立の発端となりました．

87.

Granulomatosis with Polyangiitis (Wegener's)
ウェゲナー肉芽腫症

If the kidney is involved, you are lucky to find the granulomatous vasculitis if you biopsy it; 90% of cases have a glomerulonephritis not specific for this disorder.

「ウェゲナー肉芽腫症の患者に腎病変があれば，腎生検で幸運にも肉芽腫性血管炎病変を見いだすかもしれない．90％の患者が非特異的な糸球体腎炎を有する」

Obviously the name of this disease suggests that there is a granulomatous component to it. However, the presence of these lesions is very much scattered, and one may not in fact appreciate granulomas in association with a necrotizing vasculitis in biopsy specimens. C-ANCA correlates with antiproteinase-3 antibodies in the appreciable majority.

この疾患の名前は，明らかに肉芽腫の要素があることを示唆しています．しかし，肉芽腫病変は散らばって存在するため，生検組織において壊死性血管炎を伴った肉芽腫を実際に確認できないことがあります．多くの患者で確認できるC-ANCAは，抗プロテアーゼ3（PR3）抗体と関係があります．

METABOLIC DISORDERS
代謝性疾患

88.

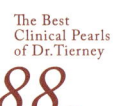

Acromegaly
先端巨大症

Performing a "wallet biopsy" is the least expensive way to make this diagnosis.

「"財布生検"の施行は最も費用のかからない先端巨大症の診断法である」

 Acromegaly is characterized by numerous changes in the physical appearance, particularly macrognathia and coarsening of the facial features. These occur slowly, and may not be noticed by family members. By simply asking the patient to look at his driver's license, on which nearly everyone has a picture dating back a few years, the change will be immediately obvious. This "noninvasive procedure" may be helpful in a variety of other conditions as well.

 先端巨大症は数多くの身体の外観の変化を特徴とする疾患です．特に，巨顎症，粗野な顔貌の変化です．これらの変化は緩徐に起こるため，家族すら気のつかないことがあります．単に，患者に数年前の顔が写っている運転免許証をみてくださいと聴くだけで，顔の変化はすぐに明らかになるでしょう．この「非侵襲的検査」は，ほかのさまざまな病態でも役に立つでしょう．

89. Myxedema
粘液水腫

This is the diagnosis you make over the telephone, when the patient calls you and says in a slow, hoarse voice that she is always cold.

「女性患者が電話をかけてきて,ゆっくり,かすれた声で,いつも寒いのですがと話したなら,粘液水腫と電話ごしに診断できる」

Among many other features, seriously hypothyroid patients feel cold even in warm weather. It is said that if a patient is covered in several blankets when you enter the examining room on a hot day, that the diagnosis jumps high on the differential list, although a number of older patients without hypothyroidism may complain of this symptom as well.

粘液水腫のいくつかの特徴がありますが,患者は暑い天候でさえも,とても寒いと感じます.暑い日,医師が診察室に入ったときに,患者が数枚の毛布にくるまっていたら,甲状腺機能低下症の可能性が一気に高まるといわれています.しかし,甲状腺機能低下症のない多くの高齢患者が,同じ症状を訴えることがあります.

90.

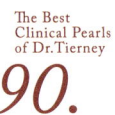

Diabetes Insipidus
尿崩症

In an adult with unexplained polyuria, inquire about a history of acne during teenage years; its treatment may be the answer.

「成人患者の説明のつかない多尿では，10代のときの痤瘡歴を聴きなさい．その治療内容に答えがみつかることがある」

　Many adolescents suffer from acne during teenage years, and it is quite common to treat these persons with a tetracycline antibiotic. These drugs all have the ability to cause mild resistance of the distal tubule to antidiuretic hormone, which is permanent, accounting for the symptom, and treatable with hydrochlorothiazide. Central diabetes insipidus is a far more challenging condition posing difficult fluid balance problems and volume swings, treated with nasal vasopressin.

　多くの青年期の患者は，10代の頃に痤瘡（ニキビ）を患うものです．痤瘡にはテトラサイクリン系抗菌薬が治療として一般的に用いられます．これらテトラサイクリン系抗菌薬すべては，遠位尿細管の抗利尿ホルモンに対する中等度の抵抗性をもたらすことがあります．この副作用は永続しますが，ヒドロクロロチアジドで治療可能です．中枢性尿崩症は，はるかに水バランスをとることが困難な病態といえるでしょう．体液量は大きく変動し，バゾプレッシン点鼻で治療します．

91.

Type 1 Diabetes
1型糖尿病

An autoimmune disease; thus no positive family history, abrupt onset often after a mild viral infection, and the absolute absence of insulin.

「1型糖尿病は自己免疫性疾患である．家族歴がなく，軽いウイルス感染後の突然発症が多く，インスリンの絶対的な欠乏を示す」

Type 1 is considerably less common than type 2, and it perhaps constitutes only 5% of Japanese diabetics. The stunningly abrupt onset is characteristic, and the development of ketosis is as well, because even trivial amounts of endogenous insulin are capable of inhibiting ketogenesis.

1型糖尿病は2型糖尿病よりもずいぶんと少ないのです．おそらく，日本人糖尿病患者の5％にしか認められないでしょう．驚くほどの突然発症が特徴であり，同様にケトーシスを示します．なぜなら，わずかな量の内因性インスリンさえあれば，ケトン生成を阻害することができるからです．

92.

Type 2 Diabetes
2型糖尿病

Patients do not seek care early due to the absence of ketosis and the breathlessness that goes with it; in fact, they may be delighted to lose weight and maintain appetite... but in this case it is not a desirable thing.

「2型糖尿病患者はケトーシス，そしてケトーシスにおける呼吸困難がないため，早期に病院を訪れない．事実，食欲はあり体重が減り，患者は大いに喜んでいるであろう．が，望ましいことではない」

The abnormality in type 2 diabetes is that of insulin resistance, and thus is seen in older patients who are obese, and indeed, whose insulin blood levels are normal or even high when tested. Thus, ketosis is prevented, but glucose levels creep up gradually to often alarming levels, resulting in the hyperosmolality causing a poorer prognosis than that seen in type 1 when it is out of control.

2型糖尿病の異常は，インスリン抵抗性です．したがって，2型糖尿病は高齢肥満患者で認められます．確かに，2型糖尿病患者の血中インスリンレベルは正常，もしくは高いことさえあります．このようにケトーシスは防がれます．しかし，血糖値は徐々に危険値まで上昇することが稀ではなく，結果的に高浸透圧となり，コントロールがきかないときは，1型糖尿病よりも予後不良となります．

93.

Diabetic Ketoacidosis
糖尿病性ケトアシドーシス

Although pH and serum potassium are often very abnormal, the serum osmolality is the best predictor of outcome.

「pH，血清カリウムは往々にして相当な異常を示すが，血清浸透圧が最も適切な予後規定因子である」

In all studies of both diabetic ketoacidosis and hyperosmolar nonketotic diabetes, while all other laboratory studies should be taken seriously, it is the initial serum osmolality which determines outcome. This typical complication of type 2 diabetes is far more common than it is in type 1, because hyperventilation causes the latter group to seek care sooner.

糖尿病性ケトアシドーシス，高浸透圧性非ケトン性糖尿病の2つに関するすべての研究において，血清浸透圧以外のすべての検査結果も深刻にとらえるべきであるが，予後を規定するのは，最初の血清浸透圧だということが示されています．この典型的な合併症は，1型糖尿病よりも2型糖尿病にはるかに多いのです．なぜなら，換気亢進が1型糖尿病の患者グループを早期に病院受診に向かわせるからです．

［訳者注］
1型糖尿病の糖尿病性ケトアシドーシスでは，アニオンギャップ上昇の代謝性アシドーシスへの代償として換気亢進が起こります．高浸透圧だけでは，換気亢進は起こりません．

94.

Cushing's Syndrome
クッシング症候群

The most common of the several causes is iatrogenic, and this is yet another condition diagnosed by the wallet biopsy or the "eyeball test."

「クッシング症候群のいくつかの原因で最も多いのは医原性である．財布生検，もしくは眼球テストによって診断可能なさらなるほかの病態である」

Cushing's syndrome is to be separated from Cushing's disease, although both are characterized by extremely high cortisol levels with a typical moon-like facial appearance. The "eyeball test" refers to the provider's first impression of the patient's appearance, which is typical, and a comparison with the picture on the driver's license can cinch the diagnosis (which may not have been appreciated by family due to the slow rate of progression).

クッシング症候群とクッシング病は，満月様顔貌を呈し，異常に高いコルチゾールによって特徴づけられる病態ですが，クッシング症候群はクッシング病とは異なります．「眼球テスト」は医療従事者の患者の最初の印象を指します．患者の外観は典型的で，運転免許証の写真との比較が診断を確実にします（緩徐進行のため家族すら気がついていないことがあるのです）．

95.

Hyperthyroidism
甲状腺機能亢進症

In patients older than 60, if you think the patient is hyperthyroid, they usually are hypothyroid; and if you think they are hypothyroid, they are usually hyperthyroid.

「60歳以上の高齢患者で甲状腺機能亢進症を疑ったときは甲状腺機能低下症のことが多く，機能低下症を疑ったときは機能亢進症のことが多い」

It has been long known that hyperthyroidism of any cause in older patients is apathetic, and the clinical features do not include tachycardia, sweating, weight loss, and other features of hypermetabolism; rather, muscle weakness, fatigue, and new onset atrial fibrillation are all that the provider may see. Thus, there should be a low threshold to test for this condition in nonspecifically ill older persons.

かなり以前から，原因が何であろうと，高齢の甲状腺機能亢進症患者は，無欲状で，臨床的特徴に頻脈・発汗・体重減少，ほかの代謝亢進の徴候がなく，むしろ，筋力低下・疲労・新たに起こる心房細動を認めることが知られていました．ですから，非特異的な病的高齢患者では，甲状腺機能亢進症に対する検査の実施閾値を低く設定すべきです．

96.

Hypoparathyroidism
副甲状腺機能低下症

Therapeutic radiation may cause hypothyroidism, but never hypoparathyroidism; these glands are among the most resistant organs in the body to radiation.

「治療的な放射線照射で甲状腺機能低下症をきたすことがある．しかし，副甲状腺機能低下症は決して起こらない．副甲状腺は体のなかで放射線照射に最も抵抗力がある臓器である」

In this case, the pearl virtually speaks for itself. Therapeutic radiation may have been used for thyroid cancer or even T-cell lymphoma of the anterior mediastinum, but should not otherwise cause the metabolic manifestations of hypoparathyroidism.

この副甲状腺機能低下症のパールは，実質的にそのものを述べています．治療的な放射線照射は，甲状腺癌，前縦隔のT細胞リンパ腫にさえ適用されるでしょう．しかし，副甲状腺機能低下症の代謝上の特徴は起こりません．

97.

Osteoporosis
骨粗鬆症

By far the most disabling but nonmalignant disease of bone.

「骨粗鬆症は骨の悪性疾患ではないが,とてつもない不自由をもたらす」

This bothersome condition produces chronic pain, loss of height, and a propensity toward fractures with minimal trauma; moreover, it has been recently appreciated that vitamin D insufficiency is more common than once thought, contributing to problems with bone density.

このやっかいな病態は,慢性的な疼痛,身長の低下,そして,ちょっとした外傷においてすら骨折をもたらします.さらに,かつて考えられていた以上に,ビタミンD欠乏が骨密度の問題を助長させることが,最近わかってきました.

98.

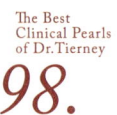

Panhypopituitarism (Sheehan's Syndrome)
汎下垂機能低下症（シーハン症候群）

Before diagnosing secondary amenorrhea as premature menopause, inquire about difficult deliveries in the past; this may be your treatable diagnosis, to the gratitude of the patient.

「早すぎる閉経を続発性無月経と診断する前に，困難な出産歴がなかったかを聴きなさい．患者に感謝される治療可能な汎下垂体機能低下症が診断かもしれない」

Often overlooked in women who have secondary amenorrhea and other symptoms including weakness, easy fatigability, and sexual dysfunction, one of the major causes of this condition is hypotension related to bleeding complications of a delivery, in turn resulting in pituitary hemorrhage and secondary pituitary insufficiency. There are several other causes, including pituitary or hypothalamic masses, but in the event that imaging of the brain is within normal limits, the history of a difficult previous childbirth may point the clinician in the correct direction for diagnosis.

続発性無月経，および，筋力低下・易疲労・性的機能不全を含むほかの症状を有する女性において，汎下垂機能低下症はよく見過ごされます．汎下垂機能低下症の最も多い原因は，出産時の出血に関係し，結果的に下垂体出血，もしくは二次性の下垂体機能不全を起こす低血圧です．下垂体，視床の腫瘍を含むほかの疾患も汎下垂機能低下症の原因となります．しかし，脳の画像検査で異常が指摘できない場合は，以前の難産歴が医師に正しい診断の方向付けを示してくれる可能性があるのです．

99.

Pheochromocytoma
褐色細胞腫

Remember the rule of tens: 10% bilateral, 10% malignant, 10% extra-adrenal, 10% familial, and 10% normotensive.

「褐色細胞腫の10のルールを覚えなさい．10％ 両側，10％ 悪性，10％ 副腎外，10％ 家族性，10％ 正常血圧」

While the above is certainly true, most patients present with hypertension which on clinical grounds is no different from essential hypertension. There is one exception, that being patients with pheochromocytoma invariably have a fall in standing blood pressure because of the chronic vasoconstriction attendant to it, which also causes the often observed pallor. In essential hypertension, the blood pressure rises upon standing.

このパールは正しいですが，褐色細胞腫の多くの患者は，本態性高血圧症と臨床的に変わらない高血圧を呈します．1つの例外があります．それは褐色細胞腫の患者が慢性的な血管収縮を有するために，決まって起立時の血圧低下を示すことです．また顔色も蒼白となります．本態性高血圧症では立位をとったときに血圧が上昇します．

［訳者注］
　パール13「高血圧症」(14頁)も参照してください．

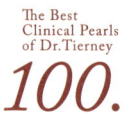

Addison's Disease
アジソン病

A blood pressure in excess of 100 systolic virtually excludes this diagnosis.

「収縮期血圧が 100 mmHg 以上なら，アジソン病は除外できる」

While there are numerous explanations for glucocorticoid insufficiency, the most common being abrupt discontinuation of prednisone therapy, true Addison's disease is a combination of both glucocorticoid and mineralocorticoid deficiency. It is this latter which results in inability to maintain blood pressure, while many patients with isolated glucocorticoid insufficiency may have systolics above this number. Clinicians cannot underestimate the seriousness of either Addison's disease or glucocorticoid insufficiency in the face of intercurrent illness, as it can lead to refractory hypotension and even death in a matter of hours if not identified and treated, particularly in patients with infections.

糖質コルチコイド欠乏には多くの原因があります．最も多いのがプレドニゾロン治療の突然の中止です．真のアジソン病は，糖質コルチコイドと鉱質コルチコイドの2つの欠乏の組み合わせです．鉱質コルチコイド欠乏は血圧維持を困難にします．一方，糖質コルチコイド欠乏のみの患者では，収縮期血圧 100 mmHg 以上を示すことがあります．医師は，アジソン病，糖質コルチコイド欠乏両者に併発する疾患に遭遇したときに，その重篤さを過小評価してはいけません．なぜなら，それは不応性の血圧低下をもたらすことがあり，併発した疾患が認識されず治療が行われないと，特に，感染症の患者では数時間で死亡することさえあるからです．

［訳者注］
　ショックに対する輸液に反応しない患者では，副腎機能に問題がないか，敗血症性ショックはないかと早期に考慮することが大切です．

101.

Primary Hyperparathyroidism
原発性副甲状腺機能亢進症

The known physiologic effects of parathyroid hormone account for the typical symptoms: polyuria and constipation.

「副甲状腺ホルモンの知られた生理学的効果が典型的な症状を説明する．多尿と便秘である」

Because an elevation in serum calcium level inhibits the contraction of smooth muscle, it slows bowel motility, resulting in constipation; similarly, calcium blocks the effect of antidiuretic hormone in the distal nephron, resulting in polyuria. Because calcium levels are seldom much above 12 in this condition, mental status abnormalities are less frequent, and indeed, when one encounters concentrations higher than this number, other causes, particularly malignancy, should be entertained.

血清カルシウム値の上昇は平滑筋の収縮を阻害し，腸管の蠕動運動が緩徐になり，結果的に便秘が起こります．同様に，カルシウムは遠位ネフロンでの抗利尿ホルモンの効果を阻害し多尿が起こります．原発性副甲状腺機能亢進症では血清カルシウム値が 12 mEq/dL を超えることはまずありません．ですから意識障害は稀です．12 mEq/dL よりも高いカルシウム値に遭遇したら，特に，悪性腫瘍を考慮すべきです．

102.

The Best Clinical Pearls of Dr. Tierney

Multinodular Colloid Goiter
多結節性コロイド甲状腺腫

The medical student's delight: when asked what the effect of iodine is in a patient with a goiter, both answers are correct, because either hyper- or hypothyroidism may result.

「医学生は喜ぶ．甲状腺腫患者へのヨードの効果は何かとたずねられたら，2つの答えが正解である．なぜなら甲状腺機能亢進症，甲状腺機能低下症どちらも起こりうるからである」

Multinodular goiters with simple cysts are rarely important except from a cosmetic point of view and will regress in size if a patient is prescribed thyroid hormone which causes thyroid stimulating hormone (TSH) to fall to zero. If a patient with this condition is given pharmacological amounts of iodine, typically for a contrast imaging study, or in the drug amiodarone, two things may result: 1. the failure to escape from the Wolff-Chaikoff block, and 2. the Jod-Basedow phenomenon, in which the dysfunctional thyroid uses the iodine to make abundant amounts of thyroid hormone, rendering the patient hyperthyroid. Thus, both answers are correct for the medical student noted above!

囊胞を伴った多結節性甲状腺腫は，外見の問題以外はほとんど重要ではありません．甲状腺刺激ホルモンが0となるように甲状腺剤が投与されると小さくなります．患者に薬理学的用量のヨード，典型的には造影剤，もしくはアミオダロン（ヨードを含有する）が投与された場合，2つの現象が起こります．(1)ウォルフ-チャイコフ（Wolff-Chaikoff）効果*からの正常化不全で甲状腺機能低下症が認められます．(2)甲状腺が機能障害性にヨードを用い，大量の甲状腺ホルモンを産生するヨード・バセドウ（Basedow）効果で，患者を甲状腺機能亢進症にします．上記に気づいた医学生にとって2つの答えは正しいのです．

［訳者注］
* ウォルフ-チャイコフ効果：ヨードの大量摂取で甲状腺ホルモンの分泌抑制が起こること．

TOXINS

中毒

103.

Acetaminophen Poisoning
アセトアミノフェン中毒

Don't forget childhood overdose, especially in the second-born; the taller and older sibling may reach the medicine cabinet more easily and feed the pills to the unknowing second child, who suffers the severe hepatotoxicity.

「小児の薬剤の過量服用は，特に第2子でそれを忘れてはいけない．背が高い年上の兄弟は容易に薬箱に手が届くため，何も知らない弟妹に錠剤を飲ませてしまうかもしれない．その子は重篤な肝毒性をこうむる」

In all emergency room overdoses, at any age, the clinician should immediately obtain a serum acetaminophen level. Treatment must be instituted before the clinical evidence of hepatic necrosis is present, and indeed, such patients have among the highest transaminase levels in all of clinical medicine. Some patients know of acetaminophen's toxic potential, but many over-the-counter remedies contain it without it being known by the purchaser.

救命救急室のすべての薬剤中毒において，患者の年齢に関係なく，医師は血清アセトアミノフェン濃度を直ちに測定すべきです．アセトアミノフェン中毒では臨床的な肝壊死の徴候が認められる前から，治療を開始しなくてはいけません．実際に，アセトアミノフェン中毒の患者は，臨床医学上，最も高いトランスアミナーゼ値を示します．患者の一部は，アセトアミノフェンの潜在的な毒性を知っています．しかし，薬局で購入可能な薬がアセトアミノフェンを含有していることがありますが，購入者はそのことを知りません．

104.
Arsenic Poisoning
ヒ素中毒

Suspect this in a widowed woman with psychiatric problems whose previous husband or husbands have died of unknown cause.

「以前の夫，もしくは夫たちが原因不明のまま亡くなった精神疾患を有する未亡人ではヒ素中毒を疑う」

Arsenic, present in insecticides, is commonly used for suicidal or homicidal attempts. There are two syndromes, one acute, the other more chronic. A high index of suspicion is necessary, because it is typical that the clinician cannot believe that an older widow would have willfully poisoned her husband. The famous American film "Arsenic and Old Lace" shows this to great effect in the film, and indeed, is not far from the truth.

ヒ素は殺虫剤に含まれ，自殺，もしくは殺人によく用いられます．ヒ素中毒には，急性と慢性の2つの症候群があります．ヒ素中毒は強く疑うことが必要なのです．なぜなら，老いた寡婦が夫を殺そうと毒を盛っていた可能性など，医師には全く思いもよらないことですから．有名な米国映画「毒薬と老嬢」は，フィルムのなかでこのことを効果的に表しています．実際に，これは真実からかけ離れたものではないのです．

105.

Digitalis Poisoning
ジギタリス中毒

The cause of the highest levels of serum potassium encountered in clinical medicine.

「臨床医学において極度の高カリウム血症を示すのはジギタリス中毒である」

One of the pharmacologic effects of the digitalis glycosides is inhibition of the Na-K ATPase pump, which blocks transport of potassium into cells. Suicidal or accidental digitalis overdoses then have the ability to stop this function throughout the body, resulting in extreme elevations of serum potassium, which are immediately reversible by digoxin-specific antibodies. These antibodies also reverse other aspects of digitalis toxicity, and may be used diagnostically, although they are quite expensive.

ジギタリス配糖体の1つの薬理学的作用に，カリウムを細胞内へ移動させる Na-K ATPase ポンプに対する阻害作用があります．自殺目的，もしくは偶発的にジギタリスを過量に服用した場合，体のすべての Na-K ATPase ポンプが阻害され，結果的に極度の高カリウム血症となります．これはジゴキシン特異的抗体で，すぐに補正できます．この抗体はほかのジギタリス毒性の問題も補正し，診断的目的でも使用されますが，とても高価です．

106.

Cyanide Poisoning
シアン化合物中毒

In a patient brought in from a theater fire with lactic acidosis, the diagnosis is cyanide poisoning.

「劇場の火事から搬送された患者に乳酸アシドーシスを認めたら，診断はシアン化合物中毒である」

Many theaters have seats which, if they catch fire, have products of combustion that include cyanide. Cyanide shuts down all aerobic metabolism, and therefore produces profound lactic acidosis. It is noted that the breath may have an odor of almonds, but this is appreciated in less than half of patients.

多くの劇場には，火事で燃焼したときにシアン化合物を含む物質を発生する，多くの座席があります．シアン化合物はすべての好気性代謝を停止させ，著明な乳酸アシドーシスを示します．呼気にアーモンド臭がするかもしれませんが，これは半数以下の患者にしか認めません．

107.

Isoniazid Poisoning
イソニアジド中毒

Many patients receiving this drug have mild elevation of aminotransferases; this does not require discontinuation of the drug, but clinical hepatitis does.

「イソニアジド内服中の多くの患者が軽度のアミノトランスフェラーゼ上昇を呈する．すぐに薬剤を中止する必要はないが，臨床的肝炎を呈した場合は中止する」

If tested for AST and ALT during treatment, many patients will show a slight elevation of these enzymes. However, if the patient is asymptomatic, it is unnecessary to stop the drug. That tiny percentage who develop clinical hepatitis often have a prodrome of nausea and will show hepatic tenderness upon examination; this is the time to discontinue the medication.

イソニアジドによる治療中にAST, ALTを測定すると，多くの患者が軽度上昇を示します．しかし，患者が無症状ならば，中止の必要はありません．数％の患者が，嘔気による前駆症状を呈し，診察で肝臓の圧痛を認める臨床的肝炎になります．このときはイソニアジドの投与を中止します．

108.

Lead Poisoning
鉛中毒

Virtually the only disorder in medicine in which coarse basophilic stippling is seen on all red cells on the peripheral blood smear; unfortunately, this is not appreciated on automated blood counts, which are in widespread use today.

「事実上,末梢血スメアのすべての赤血球に粗粒状の好塩基性斑点を呈する医学上の唯一の疾患は鉛中毒である.残念ながら,今日広く用いられる自動血球計数装置では認識されない」

Lead intoxication, once more common in children exposed to paint in homes built before 1970, has a wide spectrum of clinical abnormalities, but is perhaps best known for the basophilic stippling which appears on inspection of the Wright's stain of peripheral blood. This is yet another reason, among many, why clinicians should look at the peripheral blood of all of their patients before concluding that an evaluation is complete.

かつて,1970年以前に建てられた家に用いられたペンキによって,多くの子どもたちが曝露された鉛中毒は,幅広い臨床的異常を呈します.しかし,鉛中毒では,末梢血スメアのライト(Wright)染色の観察で認められる,好塩基性斑点が最もよく知られているでしょう.医師はすべての患者の評価を終え,結論を出す前に,末梢血スメアを観察すべきです.これは医師がそうすべき,数ある理由のうちの1つを示しているのです.

109.

Lithium Poisoning
リチウム中毒

The metabolism of lithium is identical to that of sodium, so that levels may rise on a stable dose in volume-depleted states; an overdose is unnecessary to produce toxicity.

「リチウム代謝はナトリウム代謝と同じである．一定量服用下でも循環血液量減少時には血中濃度が上昇することがある．過量投与なしにリチウム中毒が起こる」

Lithium is a small cation similar to sodium, and in states of hypovolemia, which may or may not be pathologic, it has increased absorption in the proximal convoluted tubule. This means that patients who are receiving the drug may be at risk for toxicity in hot weather or after vigorous exercise, in addition to pathologic states that cause blood volume depletion, even without a change in the dosage.

リチウムはナトリウムと同様に小さな陽イオンで，病的であっても，病的でなくても，循環血液量減少時には，近位曲尿細管でのリチウムの再吸収が亢進します．このことは，リチウム内服中の患者が投与量の変更なしに，暑い天候，もしくは活発な運動後，加えて循環血液量減少による病的状態によって，リチウム中毒の危険性を有していることを意味します．

110.

Salicylate Poisoning
サリチル酸中毒

A cause of the famous "triple ripple" in electrolytes: gap acidosis, contraction alkalosis, and respiratory alkalosis.

「サリチル酸中毒は電解質における有名な"3つの波紋"の原因である．ギャップ・アシドーシス，コントラクション・アルカローシス，呼吸性アルカローシス」

The effects of high doses of salicylates are complicated, but it clearly increases the respiratory rate independent of its effect of increasing the anion gap as part of a metabolic acidosis. In addition, and in particular in accidental overdose in children, volume depletion from vomiting may be present, resulting in yet a third acid-based disturbance, a contraction alkalosis.

　高用量のサリチル酸の作用は複雑です．しかし，代謝性アシドーシスにおけるアニオンギャップ増大への代償とは独立した，明らかな呼吸数の増加（呼吸性アルカローシス）が存在します．加えて，特に，小児の偶発的な過量服用では，嘔吐による循環血液量減少があり，さらなる3番目の酸-塩基平衡障害のコントラクション・アルカローシス（代謝性アルカローシス）が起こります．

［訳者注］
　ギャップ・アシドーシスはアニオンギャップ増大の代謝性アシドーシスのことです．嘔吐は胃酸を体外へ出し，嘔吐による循環血液量減少はHCO_3^-の尿細管での再吸収を亢進させ，起こった代謝性アルカローシスを維持します．混合性酸-塩基平衡障害は最高3つまでの組み合わせです．なぜなら，呼吸性アルカローシスと呼吸性アシドーシスは同時には起こりえないからです．

CONGENITAL
先天性疾患

111.

Wilson's Disease
ウイルソン病

In a patient who develops "Parkinson's disease" before the age of 40, look for Kayser-Fleischer rings; they are present in 100% of cases of neurological Wilson's disease.

「40歳以前にパーキンソン病を発症した患者では,カイザー・フライシャー環を探しなさい.それは神経学的徴候を有するウイルソン病全員でみつかる」

The neurological manifestations of Wilson's disease are remarkably similar to those encountered in Parkinson's disease, and before a clinician assumes the latter is the diagnosis, it is wise to have an ophthalmologist look for Kaiser-Fleischer rings. These are found in all patients with neurological Wilson's, but in a smaller percentage of those whose abnormalities are confined to the liver.

ウイルソン病の神経学的徴候は,パーキンソン病の神経学的徴候に酷似します.医師にとってパーキンソン病が診断だと考える前に,眼科医にカイザー・フライシャー環を探してもらうよう依頼するのが賢明です.カイザー・フライシャー環は神経学的徴候を有するウイルソン病全員にみつかります.しかし,ごく少数の患者では肝臓にのみ異常があります.

112.

Acid Maltase Deficiency
ポンペ病(Pompe Disease)

Sometimes referred to as Pompe disease, this may be misdiagnosed as an acquired proximal myopathy in young adults.

「ときにポンペ病かと考慮しなさい.ポンペ病が若年者において後天的近位筋障害と誤診されていることがある」

A glycogen storage disease, this abnormality may present in adulthood as weakness of the proximal muscles of the arms and legs. As such, it resembles a number of other conditions, particularly inflammatory myopathies such as polymyositis. Because muscle biopsies in adults do not commonly stain for glycogen, and may have crush artifact resembling inflammation in preparation, an inaccurate diagnosis may be made and unwarranted treatment with steroids and other immunosuppressives initiated.

グリコーゲン蓄積症,この異常は成人の上下肢の近位筋の筋力低下を呈します.同様に,グリコーゲン蓄積症は,ほかの多くの疾患に類似します.特に,多発筋炎のような炎症性筋炎に似ています.通常,成人の筋生検組織ではグリコーゲンを染めません.標本において圧挫による変化が炎症のように見えることがあり,誤った診断がなされ,必要のないステロイド,ほかの免疫抑制薬による治療が開始されてしまうことがあります.

113.
Cor Triatriatum
三心房心

Along with mitral stenosis and left atrial myxoma, one of the three causes of inflow obstruction to the left ventricle.

「僧帽弁狭窄と左房粘液腫に加え，左室への血液流入を障害する3つの原因の1つが三心房心である」

    Although this is a congenital disease, it consists of a fibrous septum which traverses the left atrium, causing impaired ability to fill the left ventricle. The name is apt insofar as it creates the anatomic impression that there are three atria. This may remain asymptomatic until adulthood, when typically, pulmonary hypertension and even right heart failure may develop, although the other physical signs of valvular disease and myxoma are absent.

    三心房心は先天性疾患ですが，左心房を横切る線維性中隔からなり，左室へ血液を満たす能力が障害されています．三心房心という名前は，3つ心房があるという解剖学的印象をもたらしがちです．三心房心は成人まで症状を示しません．典型的には，弁膜症（僧帽弁狭窄），粘液腫の身体的徴候がないのに，肺高血圧症，さらに右心不全さえ起こることがあります．

114.

Huntington's Disease
ハンチントン舞踏病

Along with Sydenham's chorea, one of the two major causes of this particular movement disorder, which in a tragic irony disappears entirely during sleep.

「シデナム舞踏病に加え,ハンチントン舞踏病は痛ましく,皮肉にも睡眠中には症状が全くない独特な運動障害の2つの原因の1つである.」

This is the first of the diseases for which a specific genetic abnormality has been discovered, and may be tested for easily, being an autosomal dominant with complete penetrance; though congenital, onset of symptoms occurs in early middle age, the first changes often being behavioral.

ハンチントン舞踏病は特異的な遺伝子異常が見つかった最初の疾患です.検査自体は容易で,完全に浸透する常染色体優性遺伝です.先天性疾患ですが,症状は中年初期に始まります.最初の変化で多いのは,行動の変化です.

115.

Hemochromatosis
ヘモクロマトーシス

Identify this disease before cirrhosis sets in: this is the way to prevent the feared hepatocellular carcinoma.

「肝硬変になる前にヘモクロマトーシスを認識しなさい．おそろしい肝細胞癌を防ぐ方法である」

Hemochromatosis, which is to be distinguished from hemosiderosis, is a disease caused by a single-point mutation resulting in indiscriminate iron absorption and its storage in parenchymal cells rather than in the RE system. When deposited over a lifetime in the liver, it causes cirrhosis, and this in turn predisposes to hepatocellular carcinoma, the commonest cause of death in this disease.

ヘモクロマトーシスはヘモジデローシスとは区別され，1つの点変異によって引き起こされる鉄の不適切な吸収増加です．細網内皮系よりも実質細胞に鉄が貯留します．年を経て肝臓に鉄が沈着すると肝硬変になり，この疾患の死亡原因として最も多い，肝細胞癌が発症しやすくなる素因になります．

116.

Homocystinemia
高ホモシスチン血症

In a young person with an unprovoked deep venous thrombosis and a peculiar funduscopic exam, this is your diagnosis.

「理由のない深部静脈血栓症を示し，独特の眼底所見を呈する若い患者では高ホモシスチン血症が診断である」

Patients who are homozygotes for this condition have hypercoagulability, the basis for which is not well understood. They also have dislocated lenses in the eye, making the examination of the fundus look as though one is looking through the wrong end of a telescope, with optic disks and vessels appearing microscopic.

高ホモシスチン血症のホモ接合体患者では過凝固を示します．根拠はよくわかっていません．また，患者は水晶体偏位をきたし，眼底検査ではあたかも望遠鏡を反対から覗いたように，視神経乳頭と網膜の血管が小さく見えます．

117.

Protein C and S Deficiencies
プロテイン C 欠乏症,プロテイン S 欠乏症

A seemingly inexplicable human condition: absence of these naturally occurring anticoagulants results in premature thrombosis, usually of veins in the legs and abdomen.

「表面上は不可解な状態:本来,抗凝固作用を有するプロテイン C,プロテイン S の欠乏は,通常,足・腹部の静脈に早期の血栓を起こす」

Protein C and S are vitamin K-dependent anticoagulants, which antagonize the action of pro-coagulants, and their absence results in a tendency toward thrombosis. Why the human possesses both pro-coagulants and anticoagulants, several of which are vitamin K-dependent, is an interesting evolutionary question.

プロテイン C,プロテイン S は,ビタミン K 依存性の抗凝固作用を有し,Ⅴa 因子・Ⅷa 因子の作用に拮抗しますので,プロテイン C,プロテイン S 欠乏症では血栓傾向となります.なぜ人間が凝固因子と,そのなかのいくつかのものはビタミン K 依存性である抗凝固因子の両者を有するようになったのかは,進化上の興味深い疑問です.